A TRANSACTIONAL ANALYSIS OF MOTHERHOOD AND DISTURBANCES IN THE MATERNAL

Grounded in research and clinical experience and with plenty of case examples, this book provides a relational Transactional Analysis diagnosis and treatment strategy to give immediate relief for maternal mental illness.

Maternal mental illness is common, painful, poorly understood, misdiagnosed and often unspoken. For many years this condition has been known as postnatal depression. Yet it is so much more than this, with countless women experiencing a multitude of different types of distress in pregnancy and for many years post birth. This book not only covers those conditions commonly known but also explores other factors such as Artificial Reproductive Techniques, miscarriage, termination for fetal abnormality, birth trauma and infertility, and how to treat them. It highlights the true breadth, depth and costs of the maternal journey and emphasises the struggles all parents can experience, no matter where in the world they live.

Written in a clear and concise style, this book will be valuable reading for TA psychotherapists and students, and anyone wanting to enlarge their knowledge of motherhood and parenting.

Emma Haynes, PhD, MSc, UKCP, TSTA-P, Honorary Research Fellow, is a relational TA psychotherapist in private practice. She began to specialise in maternal mental illness when she realised how little support was on offer for women and parents experiencing difficulties in their parenting journey. She has written articles for several academic journals about this condition and is passionate about educating both the general public and health care practitioners on suitable treatment. She is also a founder member of www.ourevolution.eu an international network of perinatal psychotherapists.

INNOVATIONS IN TRANSACTIONAL ANALYSIS

Theory and Practice

Series Editor: William F. Cornell

This book series is founded on the principle of the importance of open discussion, debate, critique, experimentation, and the integration of other models in fostering innovation in all the arenas of transactional analytic theory and practice: psychotherapy, counseling, education, organizational development, health care, and coaching. It will be a home for the work of established authors and new voices.

https://www.routledge.com/Innovations-in-Transactional-Analysis-Theory-and-Practice/book-series/INNTA

"Emma Haynes offers TA clinicians a stimulating political and clinical perspective on the complexities of childbirth, motherhood and parenting."

Dr Helen Hargaden

"An invaluable resource for clinicians, practitioners, parents, and anyone interested in the profound impact of the maternal journey on individuals and society."

Chris Riches, *Daily Express*

"A uniquely powerful book that tackles the silence that often shrouds maternal experiences, addressing the guilt, shame, and stigma that hinder open communication about perinatal difficulties."

Richard Moriarty, *The Sun*

"This is a compassionate, wise and pioneering book. It gives profound insight into the depth and scope of working therapeutically with the possible disturbance in mother/child relationship and its impact on identity and development of self. Emma Haynes shares her research, rich experience and passion about this topic with her authentic voice, engaging with the reader and her colleagues in a process that beautifully reflects the relational and interrelational approach to this significant subject. This is a book all parents and prospective parents need to read, it is certainly an impressive, vital contribution to Transactional Analysis theory and practice and is a must-read for anyone in the field of psychotherapy or counselling."

Adrienne Lee, *TSTA(P), Director of The Berne Institute, UK*

"A quote from Chapter 1 of the book: 'Isn't it high time governments and medical professions across the world focused on the care of pregnant women, their birth experience, and the support and care they need to bring up the next generations to be happy, healthy, well-adjusted and useful members of society?' And later 'Mothers are the containers of the future of humanity – the very essence of human potential and human survival. Surely, they warrant our greatest support'. With those stirring sentiments in her heart and mind, Emma Haynes sets out to inform, educate and inspire therapists to understand and take seriously every aspect of maternal and peri-natal psychotherapy. To say this book is comprehensive is an understatement. It covers everything from global trends in maternal experiences and social attitudes through to individual, powerful examples from the author's practice; from statistics about inadequacy in standards of care for women, and especially Black mothers, through to how to negotiate the role of the mother-in-law and cultural differences in co-parenting; from an exploration of serious and complex mental illnesses associated with childbirth through to the 'both normal and natural' vagaries of parenthood. Touchingly, in an echo of 'it takes a village to raise a child', Haynes includes the 'inter-relationality' of wider society and its importance to the development of the child and the care of the mother. She also includes the words and ideas of many of her colleagues and supervisees, including a Europe-wide group of interested psychotherapists called 'Our Evolution' who meet to support each other and develop ideas. A chapter on treatment planning was co-created by that group and is a valuable jewel in the book. Emma Haynes is knowledgeable and articulate; passionate and compassionate, political and persuasive in her desire for the world to change in its attitudes and practices. She intends to transform the health of generations of mothers and children – this book is the field manual!"

Professor Charlotte Sills, *Ashridge Hult Business School,*
Metanoia Institute, UK

"Dr Haynes brings a timely and critical attention to the importance of the maternal space, within a contemporary feminist and intersectional framework. Generous in her collaboration with others, this is a groundbreaking work in Transactional Analysis by a pioneering author, advocate, and activist. Highlighting the scarcity of research in this area, the author calls for expanded inquiry and collaboration to enhance the understanding and treatment of perinatal mental health issues. Her advocacy for a TA Relational Psychotherapy as a means for lasting change for mothers, fathers and parents, sets a hopeful tone for future practices in mental health care. This is not just a book: It is a clarion call for a movement to recognise and address the complexities of maternal mental health in psychotherapy. It will serve as an essential guide for TA practitioners and a call to action for the wider psychotherapy community, bringing the core concepts of relational TA to the topic of maternal mental health. It stands as a testament to the transformative power of relational perinatal psychotherapy, offering new horizons in the care and understanding of maternal mental health."

Helen Rowland, *DipSw CTA (P) TSTA (P) UKCP registered*
psychotherapist, co-editor of the Transactional Analysis Journal

A TRANSACTIONAL ANALYSIS OF MOTHERHOOD AND DISTURBANCES IN THE MATERNAL

From Pre-conception to Human Being

Emma Haynes

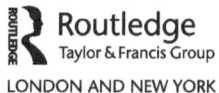

Routledge
Taylor & Francis Group

LONDON AND NEW YORK

Designed cover image: © Getty Images

First published 2025
by Routledge
4 Park Square, Milton Park, Abingdon, Oxon OX14 4RN

and by Routledge
605 Third Avenue, New York, NY 10158

Routledge is an imprint of the Taylor & Francis Group, an informa business

British Library Cataloguing-in-Publication Data
A catalogue record for this book is available from the British Library

Library of Congress Cataloging-in-Publication Data
Names: Haynes, Emma (Psychotherapist), author.
Title: A transactional analysis of motherhood and disturbances in the maternal : from pre-conception to human being / Emma Haynes.
Description: Abington, Oxon ; New York, NY : Routledge, 2025. | Includes bibliographical references and index. | Provided by publisher.
Identifiers: LCCN 2024025794 (print) | LCCN 2024025795 (ebook) | ISBN 9781032431383 (hardback) | ISBN 9781032431345 (paperback) | ISBN 9781003365822 (ebook)
Subjects: MESH: Mental Disorders--therapy | Postpartum Period--psychology | Pregnancy--psychology | Mothers--psychology | Transactional Analysis--methods | Maternal Behavior--psychology
Classification: LCC RG852 (print) | LCC RG852 (ebook) | NLM WQ 500 | DDC 618.7/6--dc23/eng/20240809
LC record available at https://lccn.loc.gov/2024025794
LC ebook record available at https://lccn.loc.gov/2024025795

ISBN: 978-1-032-43138-3 (hbk)
ISBN: 978-1-032-43134-5 (pbk)
ISBN: 978-1-003-36582-2 (ebk)

DOI: 10.4324/9781003365822

Typeset in Times New Roman
by KnowledgeWorks Global Ltd.

For my clients and supervisees

This book is dedicated to the memory of Dr Mark Widdowson, my PhD supervisor and mentor, who died suddenly and unexpectedly, in August 2024.

Unfortunately, Mark, you never got to read this second book. I will remain deeply grateful to you for the faith you showed me, and your encouragement and unstinting support of my work. I will miss your wise counsel, as well as your brews.

CONTENTS

ILLUSTRATIONS

Figures

Tables

ACKNOWLEDGEMENTS

Thank you, Bill Cornell, for having faith in me and making it possible to realise my dream of writing this book.

My thanks also go to Adrienne Lee. I admit that without your challenge after reading my first book, I would never have written one for transactional analysts. Here it is Adrienne, I hope you like it.

My thanks go to all the members of Our Evolution, who continue to inspire me on a monthly basis. In particular, those who have been an active part in my writing process and whose words are embedded within the book are Amy Lennox, Barbara Rupar, Henrietta Whitfield, Isa Delannoy, Mihaela-Leocadia Hartescu, Oliver Hunt, Sarah Crowley, Susanne Fuller and Valeria Villa.

Thank you to Ronen Stilman and Oliver Hunt for agreeing to write with me. It has been a great experience, and I hope we might collaborate again soon.

Thank you to Valeria Villa and Sarah Crowley for your valuable contributions.

Thank you to Michelle Pope and Tom Forrest for your explanations and metaphorical reflections on coils and springs. They were a huge help, and I am really appreciative of the time you both gave me from your busy schedules.

Thank you, Karen for inspiring me to 'write what I like'. I am truly grateful for all your wise words.

To Sarah Hobhouse, Lou Walker, Susie Hewitt, Charlotte Sills, Rachel Cook and Jane Skinner, thank you for your brilliant critiquing, and the generosity of your time. You all inspire me.

My heartfelt thanks go to my sister-in-law, Debs Steele, for your simply stupendous proofreading. I cannot thank you enough for agreeing to do this again under such tight deadlines.

Finally, to Andy, without your support, I would never have managed to do this. I appreciate everything you have done to allow me the time and headspace to get this finished. You are a truly amazing partner. Thank you.

1

SOMETHING IS AMISS WITH MOTHERHOOD

Disturbance

Becoming a mother is, for many, the most profound and intimate experience, full of emotional, physical and psychological extremes. This experience will be mostly positive for many women, a happy and exciting time. Yet, it also comes with risk and at a cost to women and to the infant. In some respects, the risks have lessened. Certainly, it would appear to be safer to give birth now than it was 40 or 50 years ago. However, this is not true for all women, and not worldwide. And this brings a dilemma. How do I speak about one of the most intimate and yet often disturbing and trauma-inducing experiences, for mother and child, without alienating those who don't want to hear or who can't hear, or who deny the applicability to them and may prefer to disconnect and push away what I have to say?

Motherhood, mothering and the maternal evoke longing, idealisation, hope and fantasy. Yet, these are often starkly contrasted with the realities of loss, fear, anxiety, trauma, love and hatred, desire, extreme emotion, disturbance and ambivalence. This emotional dilemma causes women to silence themselves, due to guilt, shame and stigma when the difference between their fantasy and reality is too sharp. However, women are also silenced on many levels, within the medical professions, within families, and at a societal and sociocultural level, because their discourse does not fit with the expected norms. These norms state that motherhood is an inevitable longing for the female identity, it is natural and normal, it is 'inbuilt' in their DNA, and that women should want to become mothers. Not only this, there is a presumption that women should be happy and contented with their experience of pregnancy, giving birth and mothering their infant. There is also a societal expectation that women will instinctively know how to give birth, breastfeed, and raise their children. This feels like a masculine, patriarchal norm, which, in 2023, may be seriously backfiring.

My work is with marginalisation and oppression, and the silencing of women, but also the silencing of parents, too. If I were to tell you what I see and hear in my clinical practice about the crisis in mothering, the likelihood is that I would be shut down and silenced, a vibrant example of a parallel process in action. There is a risk for me in writing this book, as I

DOI: 10.4324/9781003365822-1

share my thoughts, experiences and beliefs. I could also remain silent; I could decide not to write, not to highlight, or draw attention to the crisis I see in the maternal. Yet, I am passionate about my work, and the responsibility to speak weighs heavily on my shoulders. I want to speak out for all the parents I see: the Black and mixed-ethnicity women who are at far greater risk of dying in pregnancy and childbirth; the women who do not want to give birth; the women who are oppressed and have little or no choice in what happens to their bodies and the way they give birth; the women who have infants from rape or sexual abuse; and those who were fostered or adopted and who struggle with their own experiences of being mothered. I also want to speak out for those who identify as non-binary or who are in single-sex relationships and desire to have children. Every human needs to hear and understand the implications – that something is amiss with motherhood.

There is a crisis in many aspects of mothering worldwide, particularly within the Western world. This is a crisis that is about cost, amongst other things. This 'cost' causes many women in countries such as Japan, South Korea, and Italy to feel ambivalent towards having a child. This cost is not simply financial but also emotional, physical and psychological. It may also be a reaction, in some parts of the world, towards a deepening discomfort with patriarchy and, in particular, misogyny. However, there is a second crisis. This is a crisis of connection, or rather a continued, increasing loss of connection with the self. For some, this connection may never have been forged in the way required for emotional regulation.

In many countries life has become increasingly expensive, and some couples cannot afford to lose one source of income for the time it takes to gestate, give birth and raise a child, whether they want to or not. Both incomes are needed to survive, and so they find themselves in an almost impossible situation – have an infant and to make ends meet, send that infant into often prohibitively expensive childcare to be raised by another, whilst both parents work to pay for this. Or don't have a child at all.

In some countries, like the United Kingdom for example, the cost of childcare is so high that a couple's income can go predominantly on this, rather than on rent or even food, particularly at present (2023) with the cost of living crisis. In some countries, Slovenia, for example, there is government support for childcare. Yet in others, such as the United States of America, there is little in the way of parental pay and leave. The USA is the only country in the world that allows each state to decide whether to offer maternity pay or parental leave or not. This lack of governmental support for parental pay and leave meant that, in 2022, the USA remained at the bottom of the league tables of the wealthiest nations in terms of maternal and paternal support. The burden of this financial cost exacerbates the emotional and psychological cost that many experience in their transition to becoming a parent.

In addition, conception is now more complex, with infertility issues commonplace, possibly due to couples delaying pregnancy, but also due to falls in sperm count, attributed by some researchers to environmental issues – plastic particles and environmental waste in drinking water and within the food we eat. The shift in delaying parenting is often due to financial costs, lack of a suitable partner, religion, fear of environmental disaster or war, or a myriad of other reasons. Added to this, there is a concerning lack of general knowledge about reproductive life planning and the cost of delayed parenting in terms of fertility.

Mental health conditions such as anxiety are much more prevalent now in parents. Anxiety can be around conception, birth, or being a suitable or good-enough parent. Anxiety around birth seems natural, considering it is still unsafe to give birth in some parts of the world. I am not only talking about Sub-Saharan Africa. Some of the statistics around birth, for example, in the USA, are positively shocking (see Chapter 2). Anxiety about raising an infant and parenting is at record levels, increasingly stoked by social media and unattainable goals of being the 'perfect mother' or having the perfect baby who wants for nothing. More worryingly, and more broadly generally, there is also an explosion of anxiety within children and teenagers, as well as adults.

Maternal death has severe consequences for the infant and in far too many cases the child will die too. The World Health Organization (WHO) reported that, in 2020, of around 287,000 women and girls, about 800 per day died in childbirth or pregnancy from causes that are preventable (WHO, 2023). More worryingly, there has been a stagnation in the decline in maternal mortality rates. A stagnation that began before COVID-19.

At this point perhaps it would be helpful to share the purpose of this book. Why am I writing about the maternal, motherhood and parenting for transactional analysts and why do these themes deserve their own book in this series? Maternal mental illness is not a core part of any transactional analysis (TA) training course, nor is it within core training for other psychotherapeutic modalities. It is not much written about in any of the copies of the *Transactional Analysis Journal* (TAJ). Although we already have a broad, rich, complex and evolving theoretical base on the development of the self, both intrapsychically and interpersonally.

Yet, no matter what field we work in – organisation, education, counselling or psychotherapy – every person in the TA community is impacted by maternal and perinatal mental illness. For the psychotherapists among us, many will have seen it already in their therapy room. We all have a mother, and many of us also choose to be parents. This crisis even impacts those who do not choose the parenting pathway due to the costs we all pay when motherhood goes wrong. This fundamental and troubling crisis within humanity has in its core and essence the struggles within the maternal. But more than this, TA theory on the development of the self lacks the most fundamental foundational aspect: conception. There is also a serious lack in emphasis on the importance of protocol. Yet, protocol impacts us throughout our lives and influences three crucial aspects: physis (the growth force), potential (that all humans are born with) and intuition (see Chapter 5). My purpose in writing, therefore, is to begin to fill a gap in TA theory and practice. Considering that parenthood is such a fundamental part of human life, it is striking that this genuine and distressing condition remains largely ignored or unrecognised, and unspoken about within the TA community.

The TA community have most recently managed to bring the environment more centrally into focus. I would like to bring the maternal, mothering and parenting front and centre too, to bring it into our theory, into our conscious-ness and into our training. Within this book, I will show you why the mater-nal is an essential part, and why it deserves its place within TA theory. I also want to indicate how it can offer evolutionary change to some of the most classical aspects of our training system – such as assessment, treatment plan-ning, group and couples work. These elements are the heart of transactional analysis, and may benefit from a refresh, a rethink or a re-birth.

Within the 2023 common mission statement from the International Trans-actional Analysis Association (ITAA) and the European Association of Transactional Analysis (EATA), there is an acknowledgement regarding the need for human connection to the environment. Eco-TA is highlighting this issue, and I agree that it is fundamentally important (Haynes, 2023). However, it is not only the environment humans need to be connected to. I also see an essential need to realise that humans are losing their ability for self-connection, and for some, this connection may never have existed in the first place. If humans are losing this self-connection, how can there be an expectation for them to connect themselves to the environment? This self-connection begins in the womb, and possibly much earlier if there is an acknowledgement of the transgenerational and historical aspects of evolution. Why is this impor-tant? I believe this loss or lack of self-connection is an essential aspect in the explosion of mental health conditions and why there is a significant problem with anxiety among all ages. Anxiety disorders alone have increased from 194.92 million people diagnosed in 1990 to 301.39 million in 2019 worldwide (Yang et al., 2021). Most troubling is the level among children and teenagers. Why has this happened? Where has this explosion come from?

I see mothers all around me, walking down the street, sitting in the play-ground, who appear more interested in checking their phones than interact-ing with their infants. Mobile phones are a killer of face-to-face connection. I watch children calling out to their parents for recognition, for the focus to be on them, as it should be, wanting to engage with their parents, but the par-ents are distracted. The parents don't realise this may be detrimental to their child's brain development – they think it is normal. Yet, it isn't normal. It is a new behaviour, and the evolutionary process has not had time to adapt and evolve to cope with this lack, this discounting, this abandonment in connec-tion between infant and parent. Yes, strong words, but they must be strong, forceful even. The next generations are in real danger of not receiving the connection they require for their brains to fire and wire in the way they need.

Is it acceptable for parents to give an infant or one-year-old a phone, or tablet, or put babies in front of TVs, almost like a system of childcare? What happens to the infant's most significant opportunities in its life, these first critical years, to build its brain architecture for connection, development and, most importantly, regulation (see Chapters 5 and 6)? Is this important? Does it matter? Won't this sort itself out over time?

What if it doesn't? The inevitability of the increase in tech usage of all shapes and sizes seems to be a slippery slope. Once a child is distracted by tech at an early age, it is an opportunity for the parent to use this distraction technique time and again, and suddenly, the child is on the phone all the time, addicted to the constantly changing myriad of colours and moving objects. Wouldn't you be distracted? Let's face it, if the choice is little connection from a parent, or connection to a fast-moving, colourful and ever-changing tablet world, I know I'd choose the latter. How does this impact human connection if connection to a tablet, laptop or phone is so entrancing? It is possible to see the consequences all around us, in waiting rooms, in departure lounges, in restaurants. Whole families sitting together yet not speaking, every member transfixed with their phone or electronic device. How does this offer human connection? How does this engender support and security to the children? How does this help them learn the skills of communication?

There are so many thwarted opportunities for parents and their infants to connect in the way they used to. Pushchairs and prams are a particular issue for me and a clear example of an opportunity cost. It doesn't help that pushchair manufacturers forget (or perhaps don't know) that infants need to feel safe and secure by facing their parents so they can interact with them and easily seek reassurance. Yet so many pushchairs face outwards, away from the parent. Children have to strain their necks backwards to gain any kind of attention. Or they simply give up and lie passively. Yes, as the child grows up, they need to face outwards towards the world, but not when they are tiny. How might it be for an infant to face the crazy, noisy world filled with traffic and strangers, with no way of being reassured by the parent? This may be hugely scary, disconcerting and bewildering for a tiny child.

In the first 1,000 days of a child's life, the child is hard-wired to learn about connection, regulation, and interaction. Children need their parents to be totally focused on them, to teach them through interaction and speech, to regulate them through connection, to bond with them and to attend to their needs. Am I alone in seeing a possible link between the explosion in the growth of technology, the loss of human connection and the constantly rising anxiety levels?

What about the impact of the pandemic? A whole generation of infants spent their first fundamental days/weeks/months, the most fundamental and critical time of the explosion in their brain development, surrounded by people wearing masks, covering mouths and facial features that infants need to see for, amongst other things, their language development. How do these infants learn about speech, language, and co-regulation when they cannot read and try to interpret the facial expressions of others in the way they may need? What are the long-term consequences?

This is not the first book I have written about this subject. My first book – *Motherhood and Mental Illness: A Relational Treatment Approach* – aimed to reach a wide audience with relevance to any psychotherapist, doctor or mental health practitioner working with maternal mental illness. I did this deliberately as, at the time, I was unsure whether a book on maternal disturbance aimed only at transactional analysts would be accepted for publication. The first book was also an overview of the enormous breadth and depth of the perinatal field and how relational psychotherapy can address many of the difficult disturbances that are stirred by becoming a mother. However, I am also a transactional analyst passionate about working in and researching this area, so I want to bang the drum for transactional analysis to raise its profile and show the world how useful it is when working with the maternal.

I believe it is hugely important, fundamental even, for all transactional analysts to know about the theories I will share about conception, birth and parenting, as well as genetics, epigenetics, neuroscience, maternal effects and transgenerational processes and what this might offer to TA's four fields. Human infants are born with huge potential. How mothers are valued and supported in their mothering endeavours to nurture and care for their infants so that they may fulfil their potential is vitally important to all humanity. Yet, it does not feel that mothers are valued at all. Mothers are often at the margins of society. Even today, the 16th November 2023, the headlines on the BBC news in England is about the standards in maternity units, which are the poorest of any hospital unit inspected by our health care regulator the Care Quality Commission (CQC). Two-thirds (67%) were deemed not safe enough, a rise of 12% in 12 months. At the time when a woman is at her most vulnerable, desperately trying to birth the next generation, she is subject to the poorest of safety. Why? What on earth is happening? How is it that maternity health care is declining in England in this way?

Maternal mental illness is complicated and covers a vast network of struggles and disturbances, so the likelihood of meeting it in friends, family or colleagues is high. There is also little consensus among health professionals about what causes it, and many differing arguments and hypotheses on what it even is. For example, one difference of opinion is around the accuracy of calling it an illness. Is it an illness, or is it a reaction to societal and systemic pressures, particularly in the industrialised world? Some of the narratives I hear daily from my clients are "I'm a useless mother", "I am weak", "I should be able to do this", "What is wrong with me?", "I need to pretend I'm okay when I'm not". Unsurprisingly, regardless of the person in front of me, these narratives and many more like them, are common in this client group, with many clients feeling overwhelmed and beaten down by a sense of failure as a parent. Parents tell me it is as if they should know instinctively how to be a parent, how to give birth, and how to breastfeed. More importantly, for many women, these narratives feed their need to be the perfect parent which is fuelled by social media and unrealistic portrayals of mothers within society. Women can feel in a horrible, unrelenting bind. I don't have the answer to whether it is an illness, only my own opinion. However, hopefully, by the conclusion of this book, more of this ongoing debate will come to light so that you can make up your own mind.

Similarly, the way I approach each of my clients is my own way. I have chosen to write each chapter to highlight some of the difficulties and problems I have discovered, over the many years I have been specialising in this area. This is so that readers can take from it what they want: dispute it, change it, critique it, question it. Whatever happens, my aim is that the book poses many more questions than answers.

Perhaps you are now wondering why I keep using the phrase 'maternal mental illness'. Over the years, I have been through a few different terms. Still, I have chosen to use 'maternal mental illness' as a catchall to incorporate all the difficulties and struggles experienced in the transition from being parented to becoming a parent. This book mainly discusses the women I see and focuses on them as the maternal caregiver. However, I see single-sex couples and non-binary parents and caregivers who are not genetic parents, too. The vast majority of my clients have been and are women. For me, the term 'maternal' would include any parent (female, male, non-binary, adoptive, foster) who offers caregiving that would be considered maternal in its nature and who is struggling with their transition to becoming a parent.

It is impossible to cover all the difficulties and struggles within this book as they are simply too numerous. However, one crucial difficulty is that this 'illness', at whatever time point it begins – conception through to the postnatal period – is often highly specific, personal and significant for the mother, the infant and even her entire family. Her experience may be similar, but it will never be the same as other mothers. This is a crucial factor. I struggle with a one-size-fits-all treatment style because it continues to discount the woman, her infant, and her particular struggle, placing her in a one-down position of "we [the practitioners] know what is wrong". I prefer to listen to, respond and be with the woman herself rather than boxing her up into her particular symptoms, discounting her, and furthering the marginalisation and oppression she may be feeling.

I need to highlight that there are also multiple ways this type of 'illness' is labelled, many of which seem inaccurate or inapplicable to the mothers I see. Postnatal depression is one of the labels that I find deeply unhelpful. I don't see much depression. What I do see is extreme distress, fear, anxiety, and overwhelm. I agree that once the body is flooded with stress hormones, it can seem to shut down. Is this depression, utter exhaustion, or the body's response to the need to survive?

Research shows maternal mental illness is one of the most common morbidities in pregnancy (Howard & Khalifeh, 2020) and is a leading cause of maternal suicide (Chin et al., 2022; MBRRACE Report (2020); Knight et al., 2019). In turn, maternal suicide is a leading cause of death in the perinatal period – pregnancy and the first year post-birth (Chin et al., 2022). Maternal mental illness is also experienced worldwide in all countries, particularly low-income countries and within immigrant and refugee populations. Yet, it is rarely talked about and often goes undiagnosed and untreated. There is little written about it, besides a few books narrating first-hand experiences, although this is slowly beginning to change. There are also significant barriers to treatment due to the stigma, shame and self-silencing that occurs when women experience it. Encouraging women into medical treatment and keeping them in – particularly with medication – is difficult. Conventional treatment, which is often medication such as antidepressants, is controversial due to the risk of medication crossing the placenta and impacting the fetus in utero and its presence within breast milk.

Conservative estimates from health service statistics in first-world countries such as the USA and UK suggest that around 10–20% of women experience some form of mental illness during the perinatal period. However, this is likely to be only the tip of the iceberg, as many women say they have never reported it to anyone in the medical profession due to their experiences of stigma and shame and their high levels of fear of having their baby removed from them and placed into social care. This leads women to silence themselves and not ask for help from family or medical services. Their particular type of disturbance and distress goes undiagnosed and leaves many women distressed and anxious, often for many years following their experience.

When asked, women say they would prefer psychological therapy to drug treatment, particularly when pregnant and breastfeeding. Relational TA offers a plausible, diverse and versatile psychological therapeutic treatment which can be shaped towards the client's needs. I do not necessarily think my clients are 'ill', although some clearly are. What I tend to see is them struggling and distressed, with so much pressure from partners, family, friends and society to be something they cannot ever be – the perfect mother. Radical relational TA informs me, and how I can be with these women and parents, to help them with their particular struggles. This is fundamental as the specificity of 'illness' for each woman is key to successful assessment, diagnosis and treatment (O'Mahen et al., 2015).

TA offers a shared language that is easily understandable and useful to help clients unpick their relational deficits. We know that a criticism levelled at TA is the simplicity of language. However, in my research, albeit small, I found that TA language is easily understandable, applicable, readily taken on board and used by clients outside of their therapy (Haynes, 2019). Language can be a huge barrier, so having a language that offers connection and understanding is vital.

Relational TA places the relationship at the core of psychotherapy and focuses on the impact of those relationships, offering an environment and terminology to explore intimacy and to help the client begin to develop their sense of self as a mother and as a parent, so that they can assert their needs and address them, if possible. The focus on the relational dyad of therapist and client can help form strong relational bonds and offers an opportunity to explore and strengthen other intimate bonds (e.g., the mother's bond with her infant) as well as modelling a good enough relationship for the mother and infant. This can help the mother, in the moment, to see the fundamental importance of the mother/infant bond and attachment and how this helps to shape positive affect regulation in both the mother and infant. Affect regulation is a key factor in the treatment I offer and is often the missing link for parents, so this book will focus on this important aspect, how it occurs, and how we can help those who struggle with it in their daily lives to find positive, healthy regulatory processes that help to calm long-term anxiety, stress and distress (see Chapter 6).

I find it frustrating that within many societies and cultures, mothers do not seem to be important enough to warrant the support they require, maternally and mentally. All members of the United Nations agree that human rights are universal and should be applied regardless of ethnicity, race, social, economic, or political affiliation or nationality. Therefore, those member countries should guarantee access to affordable and quality health care for all their citizens, including maternal care (Make Mothers Matter, 2021). One principal part of this, which the WHO is currently focused on, is the global maternal mortality rates (MMR). When we begin to look at the statistics, we can see how women are not being prioritised at all and are simply not receiving anywhere near the care that should be their human right. Sadly, some countries are acutely failing their mothers and birthing people. Looking at the MMR rate helps to gain knowledge about women's access to and the availability of health care, as well as giving an overall sense of the societal and economic status of mothers. I have included these in Chapter 2.

So, here is a controversial fact. Humanity can continue without men. We see it all the time in farming, for example, using sperm collected from a single bull to impregnate many cows. Yes, this is contentious. Yet, the Y chromosome (carried by men) only accounts for around 100 genes, whereas the X chromosome (carried by women) accounts for around 900 (National Human Genome Research Institute). Researchers believe the Y chromosome is slowly declining. Currently, only women can produce the future generations. It is not yet possible to grow a human infant outside the womb successfully, and in my mind this would never be ethical or sensible, due to the impact on the fetus. Mother and the maternal are therefore critical to human survival, even if a patriarchal system does not want or refuses to acknowledge this.

As well as the ongoing marginalisation within the patriarchal system, I want to draw attention to racism. The maternal mortality rate highlights quite

9

explicitly that endemic racism continues to exist. The MMR shows a distinct difference in the rates in some countries for Black, Asian and ethnic minority women (see Chapter 2). These rates also highlight the consequences of colonialism and slavery. It is quite unbelievable that research in the 21st century continues to show that some cultural myths prevail worldwide, such as Black people do not feel pain (Hoffman et al., 2016; Sabin, 2020) – a completely false myth that is perpetuated within many medical systems and clearly comes from slavery. Most troubling, perhaps, are the MMR statistics for the USA, which is at the bottom of the table for the wealthiest countries in the world and, even more worryingly, has a Maternal Mortality Rate that has increased since 2019. Both the USA and the UK have worrying discrepancies between their maternal mortality rates for Black, Asian and ethnic minority women and those of white women. This is not acceptable.

In February 2023, the World Bank published data showing that the progress in reducing maternal mortality worldwide had stagnated (Suzuki, Kouame & Mills, 2023). The change in statistics from deaths between 2000 and 2020 would at first appear to be a huge drop of 34%. Yet, when we look more closely at the statistics, maternal deaths increased or stagnated in most regions between 2016 and 2020 (Suzuki, Kouame & Mills, 2023). Unsurprisingly, the world's poorest regions, such as Sub-Saharan Africa and Southern Asia accounted for 87% of maternal deaths in 2020. This is almost certainly due to high fertility rates, lack of access to health care, and poverty. Certainly, Sub-Saharan Africa makes up around 70% of all maternal deaths globally. Why is this important? These deaths are from preventable causes related to pregnancy and childbirth (WHO, 2023) such as severe bleeding and infections (mainly after childbirth), high blood pressure during pregnancy, complications in delivery and unsafe abortion. COVID-19 may also have affected the lack of progress in improving maternal health within the last few years. However, in the autumn of 2023, it is impossible to say what the true impact of the pandemic has been, as the research and statistics are not yet available. Both the MMR Rates and details about the pandemic are further addressed in Chapter 2.

Why are mothers so important, and why should we pay attention to their care during pregnancy and postnatally? What actually is maternal mental illness, and why am I writing about it? In all honesty, I am staggered that in the 21st century, modern society still denigrates women and continues to withhold the small amount of support that could be available within the medical professions and social care, just at the most critical time for a woman's life, when she is giving birth to the next generation. I find it equally staggering that what research there is on hormones and the role these play in women's mental health, let alone within conception, gestation and childbirth is not disseminated widely enough. This information could be used for shaping health care for women, and raising awareness of the effects hormones can have at these crucially important times. Even today, my daughters do not truly know important information about menstruation, their hormones, and the way this can be influenced by insulin resistance and the food they put into their bodies, particularly processed sugars and highly processed foods. This information could be taught in schools. I am horrified that doctors still continue to have so little knowledge about how a woman's body functions biologically and that research continues to use the male body as its marker. I am shocked that governments continue to give outdated and outmoded stereotypical views about mothers and continue to support an individualist worldview so that support is seen as something a mother should find for herself at the moment in time when she most probably cannot, as she is consumed with caring for her infant.

In my opinion, the system profoundly fails women and mothers. This systemic failure has an enormous detrimental impact on families and family life. Ronen Stilman also argues that maternal mental illness is a manifestation of disturbance in the familial system, which we bring to light in Chapter 5 on protocol. Humanity relies on the maternal to conceive, gestate and nurture the next generations. Maternal effects are the way in which the maternal may pass, transgenerationally, the coding necessary for the next generations to survive within the environment the mother is experiencing during her pregnancy. The science of epigenetics shows how this happens and how this, in turn, is switching on and off parts of our genetic coding, which may impact us in our later lives. This epigenetic adaptation to the environment continues throughout our lifetime. Humans evolve and adapt to survive within their environment continuously, as they always have done. Yet mothers cannot do this on their own. Within our ancestry, raising a child was never an individualistic role, it was the role of a family, with fathers and also different generations each with a different role, and it was also the role of a village community, where help was provided so that women could raise their children and still be of benefit to the community. This is called support.

Yet support is sorely lacking within many of the wealthiest countries in the world. If the industrialised World continues to tread down the pathway of the individual rather than the collective, then the implication of this may be the catastrophic decline in the birth rate, which has already begun. Already 21 countries out of a possible 195 are predicted to halve their population by 2100. The consequences of these declines are dramatically ageing populations, with insufficient working populations to pay for the cost of looking after the older generations. Professor Christopher Murray told the BBC, "That's a pretty big thing, most of the world is transitioning into natural population decline ... I think it's incredibly hard to think this through and recognise how big a thing this is; it's extraordinary, we'll have to reorganise societies" (Gallagher, 2020). It may be easy to dismiss this as good for the environment, but who will pay the taxes, provide the food and work in the health care systems?

Yes, the decline in the birth rate is also due to higher levels of education for women and better access to contraception, and not simply to lack of support. However, why would women give birth if they feel they will gain nothing in the way of support by doing so? Raising a child is one of the hardest and longest roles a woman can have. If she is expected to do it singlehandedly whilst still playing a part in the economy, and working to support her family, she may simply give up the idea and no longer bother to have a child. If there is so little in the way of childcare, or it is too costly to afford, why would a woman put herself through this cost and distress?

Why does society place so little value on women's work to raise the next generation? Why do successive governments value the economy above the first 1,000 days of an infant's life? Certainly, in the UK, the government has been telling women for years to go back to work and put their infant into the care of someone else who is normally paid a pittance, just at the most critical time of that infant's life, from birth to two years. Why does society also continue to blame the mother and see her as the problem when a child struggles with life? What about the role of society, what about the systemic failure that is also a part of the child's struggle?

This book is not aimed at being a political diatribe regarding the plight of mothers. However, it is political. This book is a call for action, and that action can begin within the transactional analytic community. It is possible for our community to place the value of maternal care and the care of the entire family higher. The importance of the mother–infant dyad in the neurodevelopment of the infant is widely known (Spratt et al., 2016; Monk, Lugo-Candelas & Trumpff, 2019; Neugebauer et al., 2022). There is also a known negative impact of maternal mental illness on the infant, both in utero, at birth and in infancy. Mothers and the next generations they bring into this world impact every single one of us. Not only in our own decisions to have children but during our lifetime. If there is a continued decline in the birth rate, this will impact us all, whether we like it or not.

And it is more than this. The theory of the maternal can enrich and expand knowledge and theory within transactional analysis as it helps us also to acknowledge the combined role of the mother and the environment in conceiving, gestating and raising future generations. Not only does this enhance knowledge of protocol, the deepest level of script, it takes account of transgenerational processes that occur within human evolution. This theory is of importance to every field in TA as it may help to offer some hypotheses on how human evolution occurs, particularly within the face of adversity, and how and why humans become who they are.

This theory also underlines human interconnectedness, how humans are fundamentally relational beings and how, at conception, our connections with and dependence upon others begin. However, humans are also deeply connected to the environment, and acknowledging this is also vital for the future of humanity. At present, theory around the maternal, maternal care, and maternal mental health is absent from TA. However, this area of discovery is just beginning and is a great deal wider than the mother. Theory around the way in which we become as humans, including the maternal, paternal, transgenerational (our ancestors), siblings, the environment and significant others – theory about the inter-relational (Haynes, 2022b) – is also vitally important (see Chapter 13). This book is the beginning of acknowledging that we humans grow, evolve and become within our family, our groups, our environment and within an inter-relational system that is absent from TA theory.

Some of this book is written purposely as the dialogue in which it was conceived with others (see Chapter 7). This is because I do not feel I know conclusively how to treat maternal mental illness, I do not. Yes, I have made this area my professional life. Yes, I have treated a great many mothers, fathers and partners. Yet, I only know how to treat each person as unique, with their unique experiences. For many years, I did this work on my own, and I felt isolated and alone, as I seemed to be the only person in the TA world with an interest in motherhood. I needed my own support group of supervisors, peers and mentors. As time went on, I knew that others who began to work in this area would also need support. In July 2021, I set up a group for psychotherapists called Our Evolution, as a forum and meeting place, so that we could do this work together, to debate, question and challenge each other, but mostly to support each other. I don't hold the answers as I cannot tell you the right or wrong way to do this work. What I do know is how to sit and connect with the human beings in front of me, and that is, for me, the most precious, and sometimes the most difficult gift of all.

I hope you benefit from reading this book. It is designed as a book to dip into, but can also be read in a linear fashion. Personally, I find the linear difficult, and I certainly do not ascribe to it. I believe in continuous evolution, that we grow and alter constantly, through our actions, backwards reflections and interactions with the people and environment around us. As we do so, we are constantly forming a narrative around how we are evolving and what is happening to us. This narrative is unique and important and deserves to be heard.

2

A SILENT PROBLEM

Understanding Maternal Mental Illness

Let's begin with some hard-hitting facts to show precisely how complex, personal and significant maternal mental illness is; why it has such wide-reaching and devastating consequences for the mother, the infant and her wider family; and the significant economic impact too. However, is it an illness? Or are women simply responding to systemic failure in the support system for parents, with a consistent lack of care and pressure for women to be perfect, not only in their ability to mother but also in their ability to be of economic value to society? Certainly, mothering and the role of the mother are undervalued and even devalued within many cultures. How can this be when it is mothers who are the containers of the future of humanity – the very essence of human potential and survival?

Many women struggle with their transition to motherhood and find their struggle shameful. This leads to silencing themselves or feeling silenced and this silence is deafening. It is also a significant problem for statistics, as women often do not voice how they feel to professionals due to guilt, shame and stigma, and many discount their feelings due to genuine fear of having their infant removed and placed into the hands of social services. This fear must not be discounted by society or medical professionals, as up-to-date research shows that this fear is very much prevalent today in 2024. The silence also means statistics are probably meaningless, as they only show those who do speak up and seek help through the medical profession. What about the women who don't speak up, who cannot, or who feel too ashamed to speak?

There is also a difficulty in speaking up if the perception is that no help is forthcoming, which is the case in many countries. The support offered may also not be the type the mother wants. Suppose the only support on offer is medication, and as a mother, you fear taking it will harm your baby. You have googled this and talked about it at length in friendship groups, and you know that medicines can cross the placenta and are also present in breast milk. What then? You may feel caught in a trap, a difficult dilemma of what is worse for your child – accepting the medication, fearing the impact this might have on them, but hoping to feel better in yourself? Or protecting your child, going without, and continuing to feel awful?

DOI: 10.4324/9781003365822-2

This book advocates for TA psychotherapy as a first line of treatment. Throughout the book, I aim to show that TA, particularly a relational stance of TA, can be helpful when working with women, men, parents and couples struggling with their transition to becoming parents. Significantly more women say they would prefer psychological therapy to medication (Battle et al., 2013; Hantsoo et al., 2017), and TA has been shown to be helpful for maternal mental illness (Haynes, 2019).

What is missing is more research evidence for using TA psychotherapy as a treatment within this area. I conducted the first small research project in 2017/18 (Haynes, 2019). At that time, very few TA psychotherapists worked in this area, other than me. Some therapists had seen women struggling, but this may have been due to chance rather than a particular choice that women came for therapy to help with maternal mental illness. For some of my research participants, the woman was already in TA therapy before their maternal experience. My aim is to research TA psychotherapy more broadly, and this may soon be possible if more TA psychotherapists choose to work in this field.

I hope this book will inspire more therapists to explore this area of work so that it becomes the norm rather than the exception. I live and work in the UK and know of only one maternal service in the NHS that uses TA counsellors and psychotherapists. This service is unusual, and it is an opportunity for TA. However, it is also under threat, as the NHS prefers their own system of psychological intervention. Notwithstanding that, TA is underpinned with a high level of rigour and depth of knowledge that makes it an ideal type of psychotherapy for the disturbance often present in mothers, parents and families.

The biggest challenge for parents is that valuable and effective psychological therapies are not necessarily available within national health services, which means that women may have to pay for treatment that may be unaffordable. Indeed, many therapists in the Our Evolution group I spoke of in Chapter 1 offer substantially reduced fees or continue working part-time in low-cost maternal or parental charities, mainly because their passion drives them to continue their work. It is truly special seeing a mother come through adversity and then watch her playing with her child, both happy and contented, mother and infant bonded together and both regulated.

I want to acknowledge that it is not only the mother who may offer care to the infant. We are, every one of us, born of a mother, but it is not necessarily our mother who raises and cares for us. I now use the term 'maternal' to encompass the mother, maternal care, or any person who behaves in a 'maternal' way to a child. The maternal can be situated not only in mothers or even in women. It may be located in 'not yet' mothers, within the social, political and economic care environment, within trans-motherhood and also within fathers and 'not yet' fathers. Maternal is also a word that encompasses an extensive period; from pre-conception (contemplation of parenthood), conception, birth, post-birth, maternal instinct, maternal effects (the genetic effects of the passing down at a cellular level of transgenerational heritage), and any part of the raising of children. It also acknowledges the shadow side of the maternal, such as maternal ambivalence, any form of engulfing or oppressive mothering, and infanticide.

For me, the maternal is only one part of an inter-relational system (Haynes, 2022b) within which we develop. This system acknowledges that humans do not and cannot develop in isolation. This inter-relational system also includes the paternal, our ancestral heritage (the transgenerational), our siblings and close friends and the environment we were conceived and grew up within. Our environment is fundamental to health, well-being and how and who we become. We all have a development cycle – we grow, evolve, change, develop, blossom and mature (Levin-Landheer, 1982), and for me, physis is inherent within conception and birth. I will emphasise more of these elements further in the book and, particularly in Chapter 13.

I would also like to highlight new research, which is rebutting everything humans thought they knew about gender, and turning Charles Darwin's theory about women as passive, monogamous and submissive on its head and showing that they are anything but these stereotypes. Lucy Cooke has written a hugely influential new book called *Bitch – What Does It Mean to Be Female* (2022), which, among other things, shows the role oxytocin may play in attachment between mothers and their infants. She highlights the research of Catherine Dulac into not only the hormonal responses that drive a mother's responsiveness to her infant, but also another attachment system, which is more long term and might explain how fathers, foster carers, family members and adoptive parents may become attached. She highlights that there is flexibility within this system, which allows others to step up and help out as a more communal system of parenting. This may also be why now, in the 21st century in the Western world, when many parents are isolated from their familial support system, women may be perceived to be finding motherhood more difficult. They do not have that wider support system that might have been available before and which may have been a part of the survival of the species.

Cooke is also shedding light on gender fluidity and writes about many species in which gender seems to be particularly fluid, dependent upon the availability of females and males. She even writes about female-only species that seem to have circumnavigated the need to have sex to procreate and may inspire humans to seriously question the binary gendering that exists at present and replace it with a wider acknowledgement that in the natural world, all manner of identities seem to coexist and are not at all abnormal.

Mother Blaming

For hundreds of years, and particularly within the last century, a culture and history of blaming mothers has existed, causing unwarranted guilt and shame.

Systemically, the role of mothering and the maternal continue to be significantly devalued. Yet, mothering is vital for humanity and species' survival. The maternal is essential in the formation of protocol, as it is the 'mother' who shapes the limiting and enabling factors, particularly in utero, helping to encode it within the infant's protocol. It is also most often (but not always) through the mother, initially in utero, that an infant 'learns' about safety, danger, relationships, and attachment and acquires knowledge through pre-verbal bodily processes, which form the foundational patterns of how to be with others in the world. These nonconscious patterns shape our future and can, out of awareness, govern our thought processes and behaviour over our entire lifetime. Unfortunately, the system is very good at devaluing mothers and blaming them for any perceived psychopathology within the child, and yet it is appallingly bad at supporting mothers.

Mothering is a critical part of life, and mother blaming seriously discounts the value and role of motherhood and parenting and negates the importance of raising future generations. It also denies the complexities, longevity and difficulties that are an intrinsic part of mothering. This leads to mothers feeling enormous pressure to be perfect, to experience the ideal birth, and to have a perfect body as soon as possible after birth. Somehow, they also need to breastfeed perfectly and care for their infant in the best possible way, and give their child everything that social media implies that a child needs. This is while holding down a job to pay for her family and be of economic use to society.

The pressure of this need to be perfect places an untold burden on many mothers, which is financial, psychological, emotional and physical. Mothers speak of feeling a societal expectation and often a financial need to go back to work, placing the care of their tiny infants in the hands of others, often at considerable cost emotionally, psychologically and financially. Some governments, such as Romania and Slovenia, support their parents by offering a parental leave system. Many other governments provide little or nothing in the way of support and assistance for parents, nor any kind of maternity pay or leave, yet still expect mothers to return to the working world as soon as possible.

Mother blaming can often be endemic in society and within culture, and it seems that blaming the mother has been most prevalent within the medical profession and psychology. In his *History of Blaming the Mother*, Fitzgerald writes compellingly about mother blaming (2020). Schizophrenia is a case in point where the blame was planted firmly on the "schizophrenogenic mother" (Fromm-Reichman, 1948), as is autism, which was seen by Kanner (1949) as caused by the "refrigerator mother" (Fitzgerald, 2020) and has continued to be seen as the consequence of some form of deficit within the mother (Miller, 1991; Tustin, 1991), although finally this is beginning to change. Historically, within psychiatry, the mother has constantly been seen as the source of blame for psychopathology within the next generation.

Lack of Care and Support

In the UK, maternal care through maternity units is at breaking point. A severe lack of midwives and funding and an exodus of them out of the National Health Service, is causing a staffing crisis (Royal College of Midwives, 2021). Midwives talk of understaffing and fear that they cannot deliver safe care to women in the current system (RCM, 2021). In Australia, there is also an acute shortage of midwives, particularly in rural areas, causing some maternity units to close or reduce their services and causing some women to drive long distances to give birth or receive care (Shepherd, 2023). In places like Yemen, women have to ride across the mountains, sometimes for days, in labour to get to the only clinic for miles around. According to the United Nations, some 5.5 million women and girls of childbearing age in Yemen have absolutely no access to medical care for reproductive services. Yemen has one of the highest rates of death in childbirth and pregnancy in the region (UN, Yemen, 2023). It would be easy to discount these figures for Yemen by stating that it is a war zone and what we should expect. However, war, unfortunately, does not stop women from getting pregnant or giving birth and in Yemen, a woman dies from preventable causes every two hours giving birth, a situation described as "catastrophic" by the UN (UN, Yemen 2023).

In 2021, the United Nations reported a global lack of midwives, with the number of midwives worldwide reported to be one-third less than required (UNFPA, 2021). It cited gender inequality and chronic underinvestment as factors in the shortage. The COVID-19 pandemic has also had an impact, reducing the number of midwives within the health workforce.

In the US, Vice President Kamala Harris recently published a health blueprint for addressing the maternal health crisis in America (White House, 2022) because women in the US are dying at a much higher rate than in any other developed country (Tikkanen et al., 2020). The levels of death within the Black, Asian and ethnic minorities are also high. In the US, Black women are three times more likely to die than White women from pregnancy-related complications, and Native women are more than twice as likely to die (White House Briefing Room, 2022). In the UK, Black women are four times more likely to die in pregnancy or childbirth than White women, and women from Asian ethnic backgrounds are twice as likely to die (Knight et al., 2020). Recently, the disparities in outcomes for Black and ethnic minority women have become centre stage, with several studies attempting to explore what is happening within health-care systems, particularly in the US and UK.

Within Europe, there are disparities among member states regarding maternal health care within institutional and organisational care settings, particularly in rural populations and among migrants and refugees. Some barriers to care are a lack of financial means to access maternity care or limitations in the provision of maternal care (Romania, for example). Still, the barriers can be due to fear of deportation, which stops migrant women from seeking antenatal care, even though in some member states, it is prohibited for health-care professionals to report the immigration status of their patients. Romania reports a staggering number of women who have their first contact with a medical professional when already in labour (almost 25% of all yearly births) due to geographical distance to the nearest medical facility. COVID-19 remains a factor, and the knock-on effects from lockdown pressures and transport disruptions have added to the challenges and barriers in accessing safe maternal health care.

Prevalence

Below, I have given a brief overview of the current statistics for maternal mortality rates (MMR) worldwide and the prevalence of mental health disorders in pregnancy and the postnatal period. I have listed them by area and by country. Exploring maternal mortality rates is essential as this is one way of showing globally how countries are faring with the care directed towards their pregnant and nursing mothers. The statistics show, to some degree, the difficulties women are experiencing giving birth, which underlines why women in some areas of the world can have high levels of fear about giving birth and why more women may be experiencing Tokophobia (the fear of giving birth). Sadly, even in high and upper-middle-income countries, the statistics show that serious difficulties remain. The most surprising maternal mortality statistics for high income countries are in the US and the UK due to the statistics for Black, Asian and mixed-ethnicity women.

Worldwide statistics from the WHO for the prevalence of mental health conditions in women in the perinatal period are stated as 1 in 5 women (WHO, 2022). It is thought that the early postnatal period is the period of highest risk for women to have the most severe symptoms of mental illness (Jones et al., 2014; Munk-Olsen, 2016; Woody et al., 2017), such as psychosis, mania and/or needing hospitalisation. These women were those who had previously experienced a psychiatric illness as well as those without any prior mental illness (Munk-Olsen et al., 2016). Whether mental illness begins in pregnancy and then is under-reported or whether it occurs more readily in the postnatal period is unclear (Howard & Khalifeh, 2020). However, previous studies have found that symptoms of mental illness often begin either during pregnancy or prior (Patton et al., 2015; Wisner et al., 2013). Howard and Khalifeh (2020) report that the incidence of postnatal depression is around 12% with a prevalence of 17%; they also report that prevalence is higher in low to middle-income countries. For antenatal anxiety, the rate is given as 15–20%, with a rate of 10% for postnatal anxiety (Dennis, Falah-Hassani & Shiri, 2017; Fawcett et al., 2019).

North America

This area incorporates the US, Canada and Bermuda. The maternal mortality ratio has remained stagnant in North America at around 18 women per 100,000 live births and is lower than the world average. This figure is quite surprising as North America is considered a high-income area with three rich nations.

In 2018 the rate in the US for maternal deaths in every 100,000 births was 17. To put this into perspective, this was more than double most other high-income countries. For the Netherlands, Norway and New Zealand, the rate was 3 per 100,000 births (Tikkanen et al., 2020). Statistics from the Organisation for Economic Cooperation and Development (OECD) in 2019 showed the US had the highest rates of maternal mortality in the developed world (OECD, 2021). The four countries with higher rates in 2019 were Columbia (50.7 women per 100,000 live births), Latvia (37.6 women per 100,000 live births), Mexico (34.2 women per 100,000 live births) and Costa Rica (20.2 women per 100,000 live births) (OECD, 2022). Unfortunately, more recent statistics show that the rates have increased in the US from 20.1 in 2019 to 23.2 per 100,000 live birthing people in 2020, an alarming jump in only one year, which may be due to the impact of COVID-19 (Hoyert, 2020).

The US also has an undersupply of care providers in the maternity sector and does not have a comprehensive postpartum support system. In 2019, in a report by UNICEF analysing maternity leave rates, the US was at the bottom of the table, as it offered no national paid leave (Chzhen, Gromada & Rees, 2019). Black women in the US are three times more likely to die during childbirth (White House Briefing Room, 2022). However, the rate of pregnancy-related deaths for Black women is three to four times higher than for White women (Hoyert, 2020; Omeish & Kiernan, 2020). The White House has recently published the *White House Blueprint for Addressing the Maternal Health Crisis* (June 2022), acknowledging that women in the US are dying at a higher rate from pregnancy-related causes than in any other developed nation, but also stating how much higher the risk is for Black women and Native American women. There is a plan to address the crisis, yet it also relies on the government and society to play their part and become part of the resolution.

Why are Black women more at risk? According to the Centers for Disease Control and Prevention (CDC), this is due to racial disparity:

- Variations in quality health care
- Underlying chronic conditions
- Structural racism
- Implicit bias.

These four factors prevent women from racial and ethnic minorities from gaining opportunities for their emotional, physical and economic health that are fair and accessible (CDC, 2022).

The prevalence for postnatal depression in the United States is given as 1 in 8 women (CDC, 2020), and of these women, over half were not treated. Difficulties arise because depression and anxiety are often conflated, so statistics are unclear. Liu, Erdei and Mittal (2021) surveyed 1,000 women across the United States in 2020: 36% of pregnant and postpartum women spoke of symptoms of depression and 22% spoke of symptoms of generalised anxiety due to the COVID-19 pandemic. However, the various statistics of different research groups make it difficult to know the true prevalence of maternal mental illness in the US.

In Canada, around 23% of women reported symptoms of depression or anxiety in the postpartum period (Statistics Canada, 2019). It is also reported that a third of mothers with postnatal mental illness had previously been diagnosed with mental illness.

Europe

Europe is a vast area with real economic disparity. Some countries are relatively poor, and others, particularly those within the European Union, are considered high-income. Within European law, there is a human right to maternal health; and combatting poverty and promoting social inclusion are part of the core values of the present European Union Commission (European Union priorities for 2019–24). Yet, these legal instruments belie some of the many obstacles that produce barriers restricting women's access to the maternal health care they should receive.

In particular, there are disparities among EU member states regarding maternal health care (Make Mothers Matter, 2021), especially in rural populations and among migrants and refugees. Some barriers are the lack of financial means to access maternity care and limitations in the provision of maternal care. Many refugees fear deportation, which stops them from seeking antenatal care, even though in some member states it is prohibited for health-care professionals to report the immigration status of their patients. COVID-19 is undoubtedly also a factor, with lockdown pressures and transport disruptions causing even more challenges and barriers in accessing safe maternal health care.

Within the UK, Black and Asian women are at much greater risk of dying during pregnancy. Statistics from the 2020 MBRRACE-UK, Saving Lives, Improving Mothers' Care, report show that Black women are four times more likely to die in pregnancy (34/100,000), mixed ethnicity women are three times more likely to die (25/100,000), and Asian women are twice as likely to die (15/100,000) than white women (8/100,000).

Within France, mortality among migrant women is around 2.5 times higher than among women who were born in France. Women who migrated from Sub-Saharan Africa are 3.5 times more likely to die within the maternal period than those born in France.

In a cross-sectional study of five European countries over the third wave of the COVID-19 pandemic (Belgium, Norway, Switzerland, the Netherlands and the UK), Tauqeer and associates (2023) found the prevalence of symptoms of major depressive disorder in pregnancy was 16.1% and in women up to three months postpartum was 17%. Prevalence for symptoms of generalised anxiety was 30.3% for pregnant women and 34% for postpartum women. They found that 17.3% of pregnant women had moderate to severe generalised anxiety, with a slightly higher figure of 17.7% for postpartum women. Spain, Italy and the UK seem to have conducted the most research in Europe. The prevalence of antenatal anxiety varies from country to country, between 7.7% and 36.5% (Val & Míguez, 2023). The highest rate of anxiety in pregnant women was found in Italy, with 36.5% of women reporting symptoms (Val & Míguez, 2023). Again Tauqeer et al. found that women with a pre-existing mental illness were at greater risk of perinatal mental illness.

Russian Federation

The maternal mortality rate in the Russian Federation improved from a rate of 56 per 100,000 in 2000 to a rate of only 17 per 100,000 in 2017. However, in 2021 the rate in Russia nearly tripled to around 34.5 per 100,000 maternities, and this was very much the same as the rate in 2001 (36.5/100,000) (Statistic Research Department, 2023). There is little detail as to why the rate jumped so high.

There are few statistics on the prevalence of perinatal depression and anxiety in Russia. Yakupova and Suarez (2022) state that the prevalence of significant postnatal depressive symptoms was 45.7%, and for posttraumatic stress disorder due to obstetric violence, birth and medical intervention in labour in Russia is 15%. Yakupova and Suarez concluded that Postpartum PTSD was widespread in Russia, with a lack of support during labour and a lack of emphasis on the importance of ethics within the patient–doctor communication in the medical system in Russia.

Sub-Saharan Africa

This region of Africa is well known to have some of the worst maternal mortality rates in the world. If we take the region overall (including the higher income countries incorporated within it), the MMR rates have declined between 2000 and 2020 and stand at around 536 deaths in 100,000 live births as of 2020.

Sub-Saharan Africa includes 48 countries on the African continent but does not include North African countries such as Egypt and Morocco. The most recent data for Sub-Saharan Africa is 2017. It reflects statistics from WHO, the United Nations Children's Fund (UNICEF), the United Nations

Population Fund (UNFPA), the World Bank Group and the United Nations Population Division. The statistics show that the rates of maternal deaths in Sub-Saharan Africa up to 2017 were in a downward trajectory, from above 240,000 women in the year 2000 to 200,000 in 2017 (World Bank, 2022a). The statistics show that the rate per 100,000 women was 870 in the year 2000, decreasing to 534 in 2017. The four countries within Sub-Saharan Africa with the highest maternal mortality rates in 2017 were Nigeria (67,000 women), the Democratic Republic of Congo (16,000 women), Ethiopia (14,000 women) and Tanzania (11,000 women).

Statistics for perinatal mental disorders are limited due to the lack of investigation, although they are now the focus of research by the World Health Organization (WHO, 2016b, 2018), as there is increased awareness of a gap in statistics, possibly due to a significant lack of resources. Also, there is a difficulty in the tendency to group countries, meaning that specific countries become hidden within the statistics. Sub-Saharan African countries have very low resources and a significant lack of primary health-care facilities and social protection services. It is thought that the burden is high and that it is under-treated (Dadi et al., 2020). The review by Dadi et al. indicated a high prevalence of postnatal depression (2020).

There is evidence of a need for perinatal mental health care. However, there are substantial barriers, as access to quality health services remains a challenge, as is the perception of mental health, a high degree of poverty and the inability to afford transport to access services (Nakku et al., 2016). Woodhead et al. (2023) found that 80% of the countries in their review of Sub-Saharan Africa had no published literature on interventions for common perinatal mental health disorders.

Middle East

There is a difficulty with statistics for the Middle East only as they are typically shown within the Middle East and North Africa (MENA) region. However, the World Bank separates its statistics into countries. By the Middle East, I am referring to Bahrain, Iran, Iraq, Israel, Jordan, Kuwait, Lebanon, Oman, Qatar, Saudi Arabia, Syria, Tunisia, United Arab Emirates, West Bank and Gaza and Yemen.

All these countries show a reduction in maternal mortality rates between 2000 and 2020. Although within the last years, the rates have marginally increased in Bahrain, Iran, Iraq, Kuwait, Lebanon, Oman, Qatar and Yemen, levelled out in Israel and the United Arab Emirates, and continued to decrease in Saudi Arabia, Syria, Tunisia, West Bank and Gaza.

Rates still seem to be relatively high in Iraq (76 per 100,000), Jordan (41 per 100,000), Syria (30 per 100,000), Tunisia (37 per 100,000) and, unsurprisingly, Yemen (183 per 100,000). Syria has seen a sharp increase in deaths within the last ten years, almost certainly due to the conflict it has been experiencing.

A systematic review of postpartum depression in the Arab region (Ayoub, Shaheen & Hajat, 2020) showed that it was a major health problem affecting mothers. Unfortunately, there are few studies investigating the prevalence and risk factors for mothers in this area. However, Mitchell et al. (2023) identified a prevalence rate of 31.5% for perinatal depression when including the Middle East and North Africa together.

North Africa

The United Nations classifies eight countries in North Africa: Algeria, Egypt, Libya, Morocco, Sudan, South Sudan, Tunisia and Western Sahara. Ten years ago, with the "Arab Spring", many took to the streets in North Africa to demand change in some of the countries within this group. Unfortunately, the COVID-19 pandemic has exacerbated some of the challenges that caused the uprisings, and there has been a general rise in poverty. However, the maternal mortality rate has improved since 2000 from a rate of 96 per 100,000 birthing people to a rate of 57 in 2017. The one exception is Libya, where the rates have continued to rise between 2000 and 2020 and now stand at 72 women dying per 100,000 live births.

Statistics for maternal mental illness in North Africa are difficult to acquire due to the lack of reporting. Still, rates for postpartum depression seem to be between 6.9% and 17% in Morocco (Atuhaire et al., 2020) and 9.2% in Sudan (Khalifa et al., 2015). Again the statistics for West Africa are also difficult to acquire and are given by Atuhaire et al. (2020) as 44% for Burkina Faso (Baggaley et al., 2007), 7% for Ghana (Anokye et al., 2018), between 13.1% (Adewuya & Afolabi, 2005) and 33.3% (Odinka et al., 2019) for Nigeria.

Southern Africa

Southern Africa covers South Africa, Namibia, Botswana and Lesotho. South Africa has one of the lowest maternal mortality rates in Africa, but it is still much higher than high-income countries. The statistics for maternal mortality rates have seen a decline from the rate of 105.9 deaths per 100,000 live births in 2019 to a rate of 88 in 2020 (Statistics South Africa, 2022). Three leading causes of maternal deaths in South Africa continue to be given: HIV-related infections, obstetric haemorrhage and hypertensive disorders in pregnancy (Maswime & Chauke, 2022).

A literature review using limited data of statistics from the Edinburgh Postnatal Depression Scale (EPDS) by Atuhaire et al. (2020) seemed to show that rates of postpartum depression in South Africa ranged from 31.7% (Hung et al., 2014) to 50.3% (Stellenberg & Abrahams, 2015).

South Asia

The World Bank includes eight countries in South Asia – Afghanistan, Bangladesh, Bhutan, India, Maldives, Nepal and Sri Lanka. Statistics show South Asia's maternal mortality ratio improved between 2000 and 2017. The rate is lower than the world average per 100,000 live births and has dropped from 395 to 163 women who die in pregnancy, childbirth or up to four weeks postbirth. The countries with the highest levels of deaths were Afghanistan (638), Nepal (186), Bhutan (183) and Bangladesh (173).

Statistics for perinatal depression in South Asian countries differ from 10% (George et al., 2016) to 39% (Ayyub et al., 2018). There is the difficulty of stigma around mental health conditions in South Asia. As in many other areas, women do not seek out or access care or report their feelings due to shame and fear of judgement (Insan et al., 2022).

East Asia and the Pacific

This area includes Cambodia, China, Indonesia, Korea, Lao PDR, Malaysia, Mongolia, Myanmar, Pacific Islands, Papua New Guinea, Philippines, Singapore, Thailand, Timor Leste and Vietnam. These countries showed a downward trajectory from 114 deaths per 100,000 live births, which by 2017 had decreased to 69 per 100,000 births. Some countries had not reported their statistics. However, the countries with the highest rates of death were Myanmar (250 per 100,000 live births), Lao PDR (185 per 100,000), Indonesia (177 per 100,000) and Cambodia (160 per 100,000).

Women living in the poorest circumstances are much more likely to become a statistic in the figures for maternal death. They are also much more likely to experience maternal mental illness. However, for some, there is a difficulty culturally with the concept of mental illness, which will impact both the reporting of statistics and the asking for and acceptance of any help provided. An investigation by Mitchell et al. (2023) found the prevalence of perinatal depression in the East Asia and Pacific region was the lowest within the low and middle-income areas and identified as 21.4%.

Latin American Countries

The maternal mortality rate in Latin America and the Caribbean for 2022 was around 68 per 100,000 live births (PAHO, 2023). The Pan American Health Organization (PAHO) cites COVID-19 as causing a setback in the health of mothers of around 20 years and notes that there was a 15% increase in the MMR between 2016 and 2020, even though there had been a fall in the 25 years prior. This was put down to socioeconomic, gender, ethnicity, education and geographical inequities with a lack of professionals within this area.

Australasia

In Australia, the maternal mortality rate was around 5.5 per 100,000 non-Indigenous women who gave birth between 2012 and 2019. The figure for Indigenous women was much higher at 17.5 per 100,000 (Australian Institute of Health and Welfare, 2021). The Australian government attributes the difference to a range of factors, including a higher rate of substance abuse and difficulty accessing health services among Indigenous women. In New Zealand, there is also a difference in rates among Māori (23.48/100,000 maternities) and Pacific women (22.23/100,000 maternities) in comparison to New Zealand European women (11.33/100,000 maternities) (Dawson et al., 2022).

China

China has focused on reducing inequalities in the MMR rate between women living in urban areas, with good access to health care and those living in rural areas. They have almost achieved parity. In 2020, the figures were 16.5 per 100,000 live births in rural areas and 15.4 per 100,000 live births in urban areas. China has invested in maternal health and has a policy called The Healthy China 2030 Action Plan which aims to reduce the MMR rate to 12 per 100,000 live births by 2030. Almost all women in China now give birth in hospitals (Coulson, 2022).

In research by Yan, Ding and Guo (2020), the prevalence of anxiety in 2019 in pregnant women was 37%; for depression, it was 31%; for psychological distress, it was 70%; for insomnia, it was 49%. The same research study gives the rate of postpartum depression as 22%.

Historical Aspects: the Myths of Motherhood

I wrote above about the difficulties in many parts of the world where childbirth is wrought with fear of death. Indeed, until relatively recently, birth was considered dangerous due to something known as "puerperal fever". Birth was also a painful process because, although chloroform was invented by the mid-19th century, women were not commonly given any form of anaesthesia in childbirth (Cleghorn, 2021). There was, and still is for some women (mainly Black women), a myth that women do not feel pain in childbirth, that it is a normal and natural process. In fact, in the past, for some male doctors (such as Charles Meigs – an American obstetrician), pain was considered a necessary part, physiologically, in childbirth.

Unfortunately for those women who died of puerperal fever, male doctors such as Meigs were also under the impression that a doctor couldn't pass disease through contagion to women in childbirth – consequently resulting in the epidemic proportions in England in the late 18th century.

Two particular men changed this epidemic: Oliver Wendell Holmes and Ignaz Semmelweis.

In 1850, Semmelweis, a Hungarian obstetrician, gave a speech to the Vienna Medical Society that to "wash your hands" before examining a woman in labour was utterly crucial – a matter of life and death. Once doctors took on board the practice of washing their hands, the decline in puerperal fever began in Europe (Best & Neuhauser, 2004). In the US, Oliver Wendell Holmes had come to a similar conclusion a few years earlier (around 1843), arguing physicians were passing puerperal fever from woman to woman due to not washing their hands (Lane, Blum & Fee, 2010).

> Childbirth without anaesthesia or asepsis was excruciating and dangerous: Difficult and botched deliveries often left women mangled, sterile, or lame – if they survived the infections that appear commonly to have followed dangerous labours.
>
> (MacDonald, 1981, p. 38)

Paternalism runs through the diagnosis of maternal mental illness. Unsurprisingly, this type of illness is also not new. Hippocrates was the first to write about it in the 4th century BC (see his *Third Book of Epidemics* – Jones, 1923). Since Hippocrates, various male writers have written about symptoms of what we might now call maternal mental illness. For example, in writing about hysteria (an old medical term used to describe primarily women with emotional 'excess'), many male doctors thought the uterus caused female hysteria. It was not until the 17th century that this myth was debunked by Thomas Willis and Thomas Sydenham, who both believed hysteria was related to the brain or at least had a psychological explanation (Tasca et al, 2012). Medical practitioners and psychiatrists continued to speak of hysteria as a female-only condition (McVean, 2017), the cure of which, according to the male doctors, was procreation, through a fulfilling sex life, and even a pungent smell, according to Hippocrates. This idea of a strong smell was still prevalent in the Victorian era (19th century) with smelling salts. Interestingly, hysteria as a female diagnosis declined after the Second World War, as diagnoses of depression increased.

In the 19th century, in many countries women were incarcerated for being "insane by childbirth" or "insane by abortion" and even for "suppressed menstruation", which was another legitimate reason for their incarceration (Pouba & Tianen, 2006). Psychiatry, a newly emerging and male-dominated field in the 19th century, appears to have been used as a patriarchal tool in maintaining male superiority and dominance over women. Psychiatry fused the rigours of reproduction with female weakness and instability (Haynes, 2022b), causing a "meteoric rise and prevalence in the nineteenth century" (Marland, 2004, p. 6) of puerperal insanity. Incarceration meant a woman being separated from her infant, a practice that continued until the end of the

1950s when a report for the WHO, written by John Bowlby, highlighted the impact and damage on the child by this forced separation, from his research on children who were evacuated away from their parents during the Second World War.

Only recently did mothers experiencing severe mental illness gain greater access to psychiatric mother and baby units in the UK; although more recently, many of these were then shut down. It was not until the *Five Year Forward View for Mental Health* was published in 2016 in the UK (Mental Health Taskforce, 2016), that there was an acknowledgement that mothers who were experiencing psychiatric disorders such as postpartum psychosis needed much greater access to help, including inpatient mother and baby units. Only recently has the funding begun to trickle through, allowing a small minority of mothers and their infants to receive more help.

Stigma and Shame Leading to Silence

Stigma and shame are significant barriers and cause many women to silence themselves (Staneva et al., 2015), which may make the statistics recorded entirely inaccurate and too low. Some women find feeling low or struggling with parenting profoundly embarrassing and are concerned that if they speak up, their infant may be taken into care (Boots Family Trust, 2013). Other women are worried about voicing their feelings of 'mother rage', a relatively new term in which a mother experiences intense anger that she feels is unexplained and quite disruptive. When discussing their rage, some women speak of heightened fear that they might harm their infant and so silence themselves rather than seek help.

Stigma has been researched over the most recent decades showing that women can feel stigmatisation also from within their own families and friendship groups. They perceive they will be judged as 'weak' by admitting their feelings. Like shame, stigma is a significant problem and keeps women from speaking up to medical practitioners or asking for help from their support networks. It means that when women finally come into therapy for help, they are often at crisis level with little energy and resources to help themselves cope.

The shame of how they feel causes many women to pretend to be something they are not, leading them to mask their feelings behind a façade of okayness when often they are anything but. Many clients talk about "suffering in silence" due to a real fear of judgement, disapproval and rejection. Those women who grew up in an abusive or chaotic family situation may feel shame more keenly than those who did not. This is perhaps because they are much more sensitive to relational trauma and the judgement of others.

Shame and stigma often cause women to feel like they are on society's margins. The silencing of women's voices due to experiences within a patriarchal society is nothing new and has been written about for many years by feminist writers. One of my hopes in writing this book is to disseminate knowledge about the prevalence and difficulties that shame and stigma cause to parents. I hope that speaking out about them might make it more acceptable for women to voice their feelings. Indeed, mother rage was only acknowledged recently. The fact that it is now openly discussed in the media is helpful, although, as yet, there is little research into its prevalence and causes.

It is essential to understand that those women who do remain silent about their experiences seem to have difficulties attaching to their babies. They can also have a more profound level of mental illness (Staneva et al., 2015). This silence is a real problem for treatment and may be why many women never come into therapy or leave coming until much later in life.

Treatment Controversy

Even in 2023, the use of psychotropic drugs such as antidepressants and mood stabilisers is controversial. Some women wish to remain free of all medications during pregnancy and consciously avoid using anything that has been shown to cross the placenta or to be present in breast milk – such as antidepressant medication. Other women say they can feel caught in the dilemma I spoke about earlier, that of what is better for their infant – being depressed and taking no medication, or taking medication and risk affecting the fetus or infant when the drug crosses into them.

The impact across the world of the drug thalidomide and the scandal that occurred once the link between the drug and fetal development was realised is still pertinent today. This knowledge heightened the awareness of significant side effects in pregnancy of some medicines. For some women, such as those with multiple sclerosis, who have experienced cancer, or who are taking sodium valproate, for example, there might need to be a level of family planning counselling before conception so that the mother's and infant's health can be prioritised. Difficulties arise due to the differing advice given or even the lack of guidance that some women receive when taking medications when pregnant or lactating.

Effects on the Mother, Infant, Wider Family and Society

There are different effects attributed to maternal mental illness, both monetarily and emotionally. Firstly, there is an economic cost to families and society due to maternal mental illness, which has been researched by a group from the London School of Economics (Bauer et al., 2014, 2016). The South London Child Development Study focused only on depression and anxiety in the perinatal period. The costs to the UK society taken from this study were estimated to be around £8.1 billion for each one-year cohort of births (Centre for Mental Health, 2014).

In the United States, there are few statistics, although research into Medicaid enrollees has given an estimated sum cost of $14 billion from conception to five years postpartum (Pollack et al., 2022).

Bauer et al. (2022a, 2022b) have also recently published statistics for the lifetime costs of perinatal depression and anxiety in Brazil and South Africa. They have given the sum for Brazil as USD $4.93 billion, equating to poorer quality of life, productivity loss, hospital care and costs attributed to maternal suicide. For South Africa, they used a hypothetical cohort over part of their life course (40 years for the children, ten years for the women). They gave these lifetime costs per annual cohort of births as USD $2.8 billion for perinatal depression and anxiety. When they add in the impacts of PTSD and suicide, this increases to USD $2.9 billion. Again, this included similar costs – quality of life, losses in income and public sector costs – to Brazil.

COVID-19 Pandemic

COVID-19 began in Wuhan, China, in December 2019 and became a Public Health Emergency of International Concern (PHEIC) in January 2020, increasing to a pandemic in March 2020. This meant many countries resorted to "locking down" their citizens (severely restricting and curtailing movement and introducing physical distance measures) to try to curb the spread of the virus. These restrictions were severe, causing people to work from home at the same time as home-schooling their children, bringing overcrowding in many homes with whole families couped up in sometimes tiny spaces. The pressure of being so closely confined at home meant increased incidences of domestic violence, as there was often no safe place to escape from the perpetrator. Remote working with little contact with colleagues and friends, apart from the odd Zoom meeting to stay in touch, brought severe isolation for some. COVID-19 also increased and compounded maternal mental illness significantly, regardless of infection status (Firestein et al., 2022; Jia et al., 2020), particularly for racial and ethnic minority groups in the US (Firestein et al., 2022; Tai et al., 2021) and UK (Pilav et al., 2022).

Many stressors occurred, including increased intimate partner violence (Campbell, 2020), social distancing in medical care (Dethier & Abernathy, 2020), giving birth alone (Aydin et al., 2022), food insecurity and job insecurity (Moyer et al. 2020), resulting in pre-term deliveries (Allotey et al., 2020; Lokken et al., 2020). Women were often unable to access health care services promptly. For pregnant and birthing women, changes were made to hospital protocols to reduce infection rates (Coxon et al., 2020) with restrictions on face-to-face and onsite appointments, which were commonly substituted with online or telephone appointments. In-person routine checks on the mother and fetus stopped.

This shift immediately disadvantaged those lacking the necessary technology and amplified the mental health distress of women globally. There were also many physical restrictions to partners and family members attending routine antenatal procedures and being allowed to be present during and after birth when a woman is at her most vulnerable. Evidence is now emerging that childbearing women found these changes distressing (Eri et al., 2022) and this had a tendency to reinforce and increase maternal anxiety and stress as those structured visits, with the subsequent checks on fetus position and growth, scans and midwifery appointments did not happen in the same way. A number of studies on the pandemic show how those women who were pregnant and becoming parents had higher rates of stress and perceived the quality of care as poor in comparison to those who gave birth before the pandemic (Eri et al., 2022; Mariño-Narvaez et al., 2020) or had higher rates of depressive symptoms and generalised anxiety (Insan et al., 2022).

Some women who gave birth in lockdown, spoke of having to enter a hospital, where COVID was often rife, on their own to give birth. At the height of the pandemic, partners were often restricted or banned from hospital environments, even during labour. This meant women spoke of feeling isolated, lonely and disempowered during their pregnancy (Eri et al., 2022), significantly when they could not have their partners with them at the birth.

Mothers I saw on Zoom during this time spoke of their fear when driving to the hospital with little or no other vehicles on the road, no people walking around, and the feeling of being in a scene from a dystopian movie, being dropped off at the door of the hospital and having to get themselves to the labour ward alone. Some also spoke of their sense of it being a dystopian nightmare when giving birth in a room full of medical practitioners in full body protection and wearing breathing apparatus. Some client's partners were not allowed at an elective C-section, and this had a profound impact on the partner due to missing the baby's first hours, and on the mother due to not having their support. Many women could not receive emotional and psychological support during labour and in the first hours and days post-birth from their partner. They even had to make difficult decisions about their pregnancy or birth alone.

The result of this was an unexpected and unprecedented increase in significant depressive, anxiety, and PTSD symptoms, with increases in loneliness, social isolation, irritability and self-harm (Wall & Dempsey, 2023). In one European study across five countries (Belgium, Norway, Switzerland, the Netherlands, UK; Tauqeer et al., 2023), one in six pregnant or postpartum women said they had symptoms of major depression or anxiety during the third pandemic lockdown. One of the most critical factors was the increased lack of support for women from medical practitioners, health care providers, and family, who could not assist due to the physical restrictions on movement.

The Lancet (2022) survey into the quality of facility-based maternal and newborn care in childbirth during the COVID-19 pandemic for the WHO European Region showed inequalities in the quality of maternal and newborn care. This study investigated women's perceptions of the quality of health care in 12 countries in the WHO European Region and highlighted that:

> Even in rich countries in the WHO European Region, during the first year of the COVID-19 pandemic, many aspects of the QMNC [quality of maternal and newborn care] – especially those related to patient-centred respectful care and availability of resources – were reported as substandard from mothers' perspective. Notably, but not unexpectedly, large inequalities between countries of the WHO European Region were observed. These inequalities were systematic in their distribution and being potentially preventable, they should be called 'inequities' (Arcaya, Arcaya & Subramanian, 2015).
>
> (Lazzerini et al., 2022)

One of the most challenging experiences for women was their postnatal care, with insufficient staff on maternity wards. The staff that were on the ward had a burden of care because often women were not allowed to leave their rooms and had no partner to offer help and support. This meant women had to ask for all their care needs from what they perceived as overworked staff (Eri et al., 2022).

Conclusion

My aim in writing this chapter was to describe some of the complexities of maternal mental illness and to question where it originates; whether it is more of a systemic problem stemming from patriarchal societies in which women feel that they do not have the choices they want regarding birth, overall maternal care and in parenting. I also wanted to highlight in particular the difficulties for Black, Asian and ethnic minority women during pregnancy and birth, how bias and racism are enduring in the way these women are cared for, and the horrendous consequences of this lack of care – the increased death rates at birth and within the first year postpartum, particularly in the US and the UK. There must be parity for Black, Asian and ethnic minority women and racism must be addressed fully. These women need to be listened to and *heard*.

I have given some of the statistics, highlighting the disparities in the maternal mortality rates across the world, and the lack of proper statistics for mental health conditions in pregnancy and postnatally. This lack of research is a significant problem, as this is clearly a worldwide problem for women. Is this lack of research due to the continued bias towards men within science and medical research? It certainly seems incredible that there is so little research on women and on female-only medical conditions such as reproduction, endometriosis, polycystic ovarian syndrome, and premenstrual dysphoric disorder, to name but a few of the incredibly painful and deeply distressing conditions millions of women face daily. Yes, research is beginning to trickle through now, yet so much more could occur, but doesn't. What research there is has not been disseminated widely enough.

Maternal mental illness is not a new concept and has been written about since Hippocrates. Yet, still women struggle with their transition to parenting in all manner of ways. Why? What will be the consequences for those infants who were born during the pandemic? As yet, we do not know. However, the pandemic caused such enormous disruption worldwide that it surely will have had some impact on the growth and development of those Covid infants, and quite possibly this might be heightened levels of anxiety within these children. Certainly, those children that experienced home-schooling during lockdown are showing significant difficulties in reintegrating back into the schooling system.

Maternal mental illness is extremely complicated, diverse, and difficult and impacts pretty much every aspect of society economically, emotionally, physically and psychologically. Isn't it high time governments and medical professions across the world focused on the care of pregnant women, their birth experience, and the support and care they need to bring up the next generations to be happy, healthy, well-adjusted and useful members of society?

3

WHAT ARE WE TREATING

Assessment and Diagnosis

Assessment and diagnosis are richly filled, information-gathering stages through which clients communicate the complexities and nuances of their stories. Moreover, they allow the therapist to build a picture of what the client has come for, which is not always obvious, and whether what the client wants is feasible for a workable contract. Within the maternal, assessments can be slightly different from other client presentations and may be complicated because the work is never with one person. Even if it is a fantasy 'infant', there is a sense of the 'other' within the therapeutic process that needs to be accounted for.

How is it possible to evaluate and diagnose women who may not come for treatment due to shame, stigma, silence, isolation and a feeling of invisibility in society? How can these women be encouraged into psychotherapy? As therapists, we must let women know we are ready to support them with understanding and knowledge of the difficulties and disturbances they are experiencing. Therapists can do this by stating on their websites that they work with the maternal and the perinatal. The more this is done, the more women and parents will begin to know that there is help. At present, it is not at all obvious.

There are complexities in this type of work, with all manner of possible presentations. For example, fertility issues, genetic abnormalities, or artificial reproductive techniques, such as donor eggs and sperm, which can complicate the process and put pressure on relationships in ways couples might never have experienced before. There are mums who bring their infants to therapy, because childcare is too expensive, too difficult to find, or perhaps separating from their child is one of their struggles, adding another dimension to the therapeutic process and needing to be contracted for appropriately.

To give some idea of the depth and breadth of this type of work, I have included the common presentations I see and also some of the 'confounders' – the added factors, such as addiction, that often mean the treatment is composed of different elements, all needing attention. I have split these into time points from pre-conception to post-birth. Some cross over with other time points; some are specific to just one. In Chapter 12, I have also included some

DOI: 10.4324/9781003365822-3

of the less common yet complex presentations that can occur, to show how highly nuanced and ethically charged client presentations can be.

During assessment and diagnosis, I focus on the idiographic (unique) features of the person in front of me. I find it helpful to evaluate the essential elements I am being asked to treat, rather than making assumptions, utilising a more universal or 'average' set of constructs used by the medical profession, for example. For me, psychotherapy is not only about symptom alleviation. It is about seeking the underlying cause, which may sit deeply beneath the mental illness and may be developmental and transgenerational in nature. Knowing how the woman is feeling and the myriad of symptoms is beneficial. However, assessment is much more than this. It helps me to focus entirely on the person in front of me and the specificity of illness – their unique experience, which is unlikely to be the same as anybody else's. This uniqueness is essential and needs to be accounted for. This is why I have not attempted to develop a treatment protocol, because I don't believe each woman would fit a one-size type of treatment plan. I also don't believe a protocol can offer my clients the long-lasting relief that I aim for. Of course, I am biased, as I work in private practice often over the long term. When working within a medical profession or in a charity, it may be that only short term – six to twelve sessions – is affordable and therefore possible. Short-term relational psychotherapy is possible for maternal mental illness, and I will explain more about this later in this chapter and in Chapter 7.

I also want to consider the differences between assessment and diagnosis, as they mean quite different things, even though they are often placed together in a sentence, which can give a false sense of similarity. I have therefore split them into two separate categories below. Assessment is the gathering of information needed as a first step towards evaluating a client and helps to inform our diagnosis, contracting and treatment planning. Here, I use the term diagnosis lightly as I am not a psychiatrist nor a medical doctor. I recognise that some clients find having a diagnosis or label helpful. Yet others may find being diagnosed concerning and rigid and may even disagree with the diagnosis. To inform the diagnosis as appropriately as possible, specific tools are available, such as checklists, rating scales and screening tools (for example the Edinburgh Postnatal Depression Scale – EPDS; the Patient Health Questionnaire – PHQ-9; the Depression, Anxiety and Stress Scale – DASS-21). These are widely used, mainly in a medical context; some may be useful when assessing and diagnosing a client for TA psychotherapy, but that is up to the clinician's choice.

One of the essential aspects of assessing a client is deciding whether I can help them and if TA psychotherapy is the most suitable option for them. This might be surprising, but I always keep in mind the many reasons why therapy might not be valid. Not everyone finds it helpful or the client may be experiencing something outside my capability; for example, working with a pregnant mum who is an addict and perhaps also diagnosed with schizophrenia and on medication I am not experienced with. A diagnosis of postpartum psychosis would almost always need the mother to be cared for by a psychiatric team, and psychotherapy may not be appropriate. I speak more about this type of psychosis in Chapter 12.

Assessment

When I meet a new client, I want to gain information from as many sources as possible to help understand what the client is bringing and what they want from me and therapy in order to assess whether I can help them. This begins with the first contact, which can be startlingly rich in information. What is the client telling me in that first email or phone call? What are my initial feelings and thoughts; what am I 'seeing' or not seeing? In my experience, assessment takes time to gain a clear 'view' (or perhaps understanding) of the client and often requires multiple sessions to obtain the necessary information about the person, how they are functioning, their behaviour, their values and concerns, any goals for therapy and a basic medical and psychiatric history, including any medications they are taking. I use a basic form I have devised over the years as a prompt to help gather this information because, over time, I have found that the level of dysregulation may be so high that this can take centre stage, pushing aside the assessment process and causing me to focus on regulation first and foremost.

Some therapists like to send a client their own assessment form for the client to fill in, along with their contract, so that some more mundane elements are gathered before the first session. Others have a form to fill in within that first session. Mark Widdowson has written a guide to what you might want to consider when assessing a client (Widdowson, 2010, p. 115). Other signs I am looking for are discounting (Mellor & Schiff), driver information (Kahler, 1975), and injunctions (Goulding & Goulding, 1976), anything that might aid me with my diagnosis. I am also considering the most appropriate and effective help. However, this can be tenuous and needs to remain flexible, as what a client perceives as effective help might be different to my thoughts.

Women struggling in their transition to becoming a parent often wait until they are in crisis before asking for help. This can mean the first email may seem dramatic or the opposite, dismissive of their experience or perhaps even suggesting no help is possible. Some don't know what they are coming for and may seem confused and troubled yet unable to say what is confusing and troubling them. Some feel so wretched that they simply want to find some form of enjoyment in being with their child, which can feel elusive and even impossible. I also receive a lot of first contact information from partners, which immediately brings a dilemma. The partner is usually keen for the mother to see me, but often she is not at all keen. She has to be ready and willing to come for any kind of meaningful therapy to begin, so in these instances I will not see the mother unless she approaches me.

The difficulties clients come with are so vast in scope, and there are so many possible presentations that I find it essential to know which clients I might signpost on. Whatever the client wants, I have to ask myself if it is achievable here with me, as I am no miracle worker and won't agree to something I cannot help with. This is important to consider. Perinatal psychotherapy is not an area where a therapist should take on a client because they want experience or need hours. Remember, this is not just the mother or the couple that is impacted, it is the infant too. Taking on clients outside the therapist's experience is not an option, as too much is at stake. I would advocate for those interested in working in this area to gain experience first through working in environments that specialise in this area such as women's charities. It is also useful to ensure their supervisor has experience of, or works in this area. Finally, spending time shadowing staff in inpatient mother and baby units can be an extremely useful experience.

Assessing the client's capacity and how they maintain their ability to function in the world is necessary. However, there is often not much Adult present (Berne, 1957). Most clients are firmly in their Child ego state (Berne, 1957), imbued with panic and fear, emotional, dysregulated and often are unable to cope. Many also have a particularly troublesome Parent ego state (Berne, 1957), which performs the role of masochistic inner critic and can cause untold damage due to the continued pressure of the societal myth that mothers need to be perfect. This pernicious inner critic needs to be confronted within the therapy, so it is helpful to assess whether it exists right from the beginning of the work and the level of criticism, which is usually high and can be breathtakingly harsh.

With the advent of online working, there is added assessment information to incorporate. This would include added risk management elements, such as their address and whether this is where the client is 'coming' from when connecting online; what country they live in and the laws about psychotherapy within that country; who their support network is and who they live with; their medical doctor (with contact details) and an agreed point of contact for any concerns about their well-being. This is necessary because what do we do when we have an online client living in another country who does not turn up one day, or about whom we have serious concerns? It is not ethical to leave this hanging, so I find it helpful to know there is someone I can contact to check they are safe. Otherwise, my mind has a habit of filling a vacuum of knowledge with fear and catastrophic thought – have they had an accident? Are they dead? Have they been the victim of domestic abuse? I prefer to shut down that particular train of thought immediately by reality-checking what is going on, so I contract carefully about whom to contact from the outset. Finally, I also need to ensure I am insured to work with the client and know who their local support services would be, how to contact them, any legal requirements and any research I might need to help with cultural differences and diversity.

Regardless of how you assess your clients, information is required to gain a clear view of what the client is hoping for and what is possible, so that a contract can be co-created for treatment. Above and beyond that, I also need to know where in their parenting journey a person is. Is it a first step into parenting? Perhaps there has been a negative experience prior (either due to a difficult pregnancy or maybe birth trauma), which is causing anxiety in the present. I need to know if medication is being taken, which is particularly important in pregnancy and postnatally, as some medicines can impact the fetus, passing through the placenta or into breast milk. It is not for me to state whether or not someone should be taking medication. However, it is essential information, particularly if the medication may impact the person's functioning and mental acuity.

Partners and support networks are usually key to the success of treatment for perinatal mental illness. I typically offer a joint single session with a partner at some point within the treatment, mainly as a psychoeducational session, so the partner can ask me questions to which they would like an answer. I speak more about this in Chapter 9, in the chapter on working with couples. It is also a useful time to clarify the partner's role, as I find that often they don't quite understand what their role actually is, nor what to do for the best.

The Infant in the Therapy Room

One element that is not usual in standard psychotherapy sessions is the presence of the infant in the therapy room. I do not always see women with their infants, as some women choose to come alone. However, for some mothers even the thought of attending a session without their baby can be too difficult to contemplate. Others will be breastfeeding and may need to feed during the session. For others, finding childcare is too complicated and would preclude the woman from attending her sessions. I like to leave it up to each client to make up their own mind.

Having the baby in the room can be helpful. It offers a window into the woman's parenting style and provides a chance to see how the mother and infant are bonding. Berne said, "Observation is the basis of all good clinical work and takes precedence even over technique" (1966, pp. 65–66). Observing the dyad in front of me can give me valuable information I would not have if I were unwilling to see the mother with her child. Having the capacity to watch and notice the interactions between mother and child whilst still offering psychotherapy can be daunting. As with seeing clients online, rather than face-to-face, seeing the two (or more) together means a different form of psychotherapy. It does have an impact on both my client's behaviour with me (and with their infant) and on me as I may have an infant crawl towards me and try to interact with me just at the moment of trying to offer an intervention within the discourse. I try to constantly monitor my countertransference for clues about what may be happening in the transferential domain (see Chapter 6 for more about this), as this can be such useful information. It is also up to the mother to choose when to come alone and this can be a turning point in her therapy. Many women can be quite obsessive about their infants, and are really unsure of leaving them with anyone, even the infant's other parent. For these women, the move towards coming alone marks a shift in the mother/infant relationship, whereby the mother can allow a sense of separation from her infant, even if it is only for an hour per week.

Assessment Tools

Various medical-style assessment tools exist for use within the perinatal period, some of which are usefully non-gendered and non-specific, such as the Patient Health Questionnaire 9 (PHQ-9), the Generalised Anxiety Disorder Assessment 7 (GAD-7) and the Depression, Anxiety and Support Scale (DASS-21). Other tools have been purposely invented to account for postnatal depression – for example, the Edinburgh Postnatal Depression Scale (EPDS). These tools are self-administered, often free to use, and translated into different languages. Many of these tools are used within medical settings to keep track of change and shift in mood in clients and can be used similarly in private practice.

The difficulty with these tools is around the use that is made of them and what the tool is trying to quantify. For instance, how does a woman quantify her grief after stillbirth, or after her twelfth miscarriage? How does she pick a number on a scale for this? Can our subjective experience be measured, and should it be measured this way? Does the tool and how it asks people to scale their feelings offer us anything useful? What precisely are we using the tools for? Who gains the benefit of the tool? Researchers? When using these tools, I have found that some of my clients simply find the questions purposeless and without meaning to them and their experience, and some clients can become quite dysregulated and emotional when considering the questions.

In the short term, movement in the tool's scores may also seem in the wrong direction, i.e. the client seems to be increasingly unwell. This can happen with maternal mental illness. Women initially find it difficult to voice the distress they feel, and when filling out an initial form such as the EPDS, or GAD7, they might not give a realistic response. Instead, they may mask their symptoms and adaptively reduce the score to what they think the therapist or clinician wants to hear. After several sessions, once the client is more certain the clinician can listen without judgement and will not dismiss their symptoms, they may find their voice more fully, and the accuracy of their score increases in subsequent uses, often causing the score to rise, sometimes dramatically. If the therapist is new to working in this area and struggles with their own level of people pleasing, this rise in score can seriously impact their faith in their own ability.

Fear of judgement is critical in the perinatal period, more so than with any other clients I see. Women are so used to being judged, shamed, or dismissed that they often feel the need to minimise and mask their symptoms due to the fear of these being denied or being seen as overly dramatic or due to guilt. Alternatively, the relief of speaking to a clinician about how they are feeling can mean that the instruments show an enormous improvement quite quickly. When this happens, exploring the responses together can lead to a more accurate representation of the reality of the woman's position. Beware of discounting at this point. Many women are so used to hiding behind a façade of OK-ness due to their sense of failure as a mother, that admitting they need help heightens this sense of failure (Slade et al., 2010), and they will outwardly project being okay but are inwardly quite unwell.

The tools, therefore, can be useful to give a semblance of progress and for research purposes within a service or private practice. However, they need to be used mindfully, acknowledging that they can only ever provide a snapshot of that particular moment, on that particular day, which may not be representative of any other day.

Diagnosis

The maternal is a vast area and includes so many different presentations that it can feel overwhelming as a clinician. With so many aspects going on – trauma and crisis causing profound dysregulation, loss and grief, prior mental illness, relationship and economic difficulties, drug and alcohol addiction, or eating disorders, for example – I need to know exactly what it is I am diagnosing when working with women in the perinatal stage.

The medical definition of diagnosis means identifying and naming an illness or condition. However, this is a difficulty for me. I am not a psychiatrist, so what am I actually diagnosing? It is too easy to say that women are experiencing mental illness. Are they? Or are they experiencing a natural transition from being someone's child to becoming someone's parent, with all the struggles and difficulties that come with this transition? How do I know the client in front of me even has a mental illness? The client may believe they are experiencing difficulty grappling with a new role in their life, one that they thought they might know how to do. Is it even helpful to speak about diagnosis? I don't use this term with a client, as I perceive it as pathologising. However, I might use it in supervision when narrating what my client is experiencing and why they are struggling.

There are so many difficulties with the word diagnosis in the perinatal period. The women I see speak of so much stigma and shame around their failure as a mother that they find it difficult to ask for help. How do I diagnose this sense of failure? Pregnancy and the postpartum are so often portrayed as such a happy, wonderful time. If this is not your experience, it is daunting to admit to experiencing this time negatively. This sense of failure is often joined by a pernicious and abusive internal critical voice, provoking shame and increasing the sense of failure. This critical voice is also very good at questioning why it is so difficult, as other women do it all the time, and criticising that the woman must be abnormal because she is not enjoying her baby and revelling in breastfeeding and being a mum.

Other barriers to asking for help are lack of time and energy, usual for a new mum and yet discounted as normal within society, with comments such as "you'll be ok", "new mums feel like you do", or "you'll get used to it". Mothers speak to me of feeling overwhelmed by motherhood and simple day-to-day tasks, like getting dressed, putting the washing on, making a meal, and even getting a hot cup of tea, all of which makes asking for help and attending appointments to access services seem impossible, let alone the lack of childcare on offer so that she can attend these appointments.

I believe one of the most significant difficulties with diagnosis is the differing hypotheses, theories and philosophical debates that exist due to the lack of agreement between medical practitioners, researchers and scientists on how the 'disease' (maternal mental illness) develops (the pathogenesis). Many mothers tell me they perceive themselves as going through a life struggle rather than being ill. However, the research is often focused on biomedical explanations of perinatal mental illness (Meltzer-Brody, 2011), and symptoms are described by doctors and researchers, most commonly in nosological terms of classification (i.e., medical science terms) not specific to the perinatal period. As there is this skew towards medical explanations, how do women who are struggling due to other difficulties that might not be medical but more systemic – such as lack of support, financial stability, and a stable home life – align what is happening to them as a medical illness?

For me, there is also a difficulty in using diagnostic criteria such as *The Diagnostic and Statistical Manual* (DSM), in particular the most current version – DSM-5 (APA, 2013) – as the actual symptoms being described to me by women may not be in line with the diagnostic criteria in the DSM. The DSM only highlights postnatal depression and no longer has this as a separate diagnosis from standard depression – it is now incorporated as a sub-section. There is no recognition within the DSM that mental illness is often present throughout the entire year post-birth (O'Hara & McCabe, 2013; Rallis et al., 2014); the only recognition is within the first four weeks post birth.

More importantly, the women I see simply do not speak of or describe themselves in the terminology that medical practitioners often use. In my experience, they rarely talk about feeling depressed unless they have been told they are depressed by their doctor. Instead, I find they speak about feeling distressed, overwhelmed, seriously anxious, stressed and fearful they are going mad. All of these are difficult to describe to a medic without a sense of being judged as overly dramatic or feeling their symptoms are lost in translation. I don't find a medical diagnosis necessarily helpful, hence why I tend to use the terms my clients use.

Common Presentations at Different Time Points

Table 3.1 is a chart of different types of challenging experiences within the peri-natal period. I have included pre-conception because it is often dismissed or not considered at all. Pre-conception includes ambivalence or fear about becoming a parent. Exploring these before conception and within pregnancy can be helpful. There is often shame attached to this ambivalence and fear, which may be cultural, with family and children elevated to a highly desirable position in many cultures, or it may be due to a sense of societal expectation and pressure that women should, or are expected to want to have children when they actually might not.

I have included some of the medical presentations in the list below because no matter what the client is relating to me, whether it is low mood, anxiety or lack of support, sometimes it is helpful to have all of these possibilities in the back of my mind. Some of the presentations I have included cover all time points from conception to post-birth. Mental illness can occur at any time within these different time points. The most common mental health conditions are:

- Anxiety
- Extreme fear
- Stress
- Distress
- Depression
- Grief
- Loss of sense of self.

Added difficulties may be:

- Sexual abuse – particularly childhood sexual abuse and rape
- Domestic abuse – this may be reported as rape and sexual abuse within a re-lationship or coercive control – emotionally, psychologically and physically
- Trauma – the loss of a parent (a motherless mother, for example), fleeing war or deprivation (migration), poverty and violence, disability through trauma, prior birth trauma
- Adoption
- Twins and multiples
- Neurodivergence – either the parent is neurodivergent, or the child or both
- Addiction – to food, alcohol, substance misuse, exercise, etc.
- Self-harm
- Single parenting
- Shame
- Stigma
- Physical illness/Disability – fibromyalgia, myalgic encephalomyelitis (M.E. or chronic fatigue syndrome), long Covid, rheumatoid arthritis, epilepsy, diabetes, for example.

Table 3.1 The Most Common Presentations within the Maternal Period

Pre-conception	Conception	Pregnancy	Birth	Post-Birth
Contemplation	Artificial	Miscarriage	Stillbirth	Mental illness/
Tokophobia	reproductive	Loss	Neonatal	mood
(fear of	techniques	Tokophobia	death	disorders
childbirth)	(ART)	Hyperemisis	Loss	Postpartum
Ambivalence	– including	gravidarum	Premature	psychosis
Gender fluidity	IVF	(extreme	birth/	Neurodivergence
and parenting	Working with	sickness)	parenting a	(parent/child)
Older	single-sex	Mental Illness/	High-	Bonding/
Parenthood	couples and	Mood disorders	dependency	Attachment
Premenstrual	non-binary	Carrying twins/	baby	Parenting a child
dysphoric	people	multiples	Birth trauma	with
disorder	Infertility	Abortion	Twins/	disabilities
(PMDD)	Endometriosis/	Termination for	multiples	
Known	Polycystic	medical reasons	Mood	
disorders, e.g.	ovarian	(TFMR)	disorders	
endometriosis	syndrome			
	Tokophobia			

What We Might See in the Therapy Room?

When a parent is struggling with this life transition, protocol can be stirred, and this can have a detrimental impact on the mother. Other things can also stir up protocol, particularly if pregnant women or parents are fleeing from civil unrest or war (Ukraine, Syria, Ethiopia, Sudan, Gaza), experiencing mass migration, extreme fear, and economic hardship. Other things to take into account in assessment and diagnosis are family situations. For example, if the baby has been conceived in situations that are culturally unacceptable or if there are difficulties in the relationship between the future parents. With the advent of global warming, ecological events such as drought and famine will almost certainly also impact parents' mental health.

In the chapter on protocol (Chapter 5), Ronen Stilman and I highlight transgenerational scripting and the importance of accounting for this. Asking about historical events can be hugely important, as can asking about the person's own birth story. What do they know about their conception and birth? Were they wanted, or were they an 'accident'? How was their birth? Was it easy or difficult? Was their mother impacted by her own mental ill-health? What about the two grandmothers? These questions help us to understand how specific script messages can get passed down through the generations. The messages or modelling that happens in families is so important – for example, those women who have a sense that, in their family, mothers suffer and become mentally unwell, psychotic even. These mothers tend to expect they will be ill, too. Some are determined to do it differently from their own mother. When this doesn't happen, as inevitably sometimes it doesn't, the impact can be powerful, causing some women to spiral into deeply negative states. I hear so many women speak of the inevitability of experiencing the same as their mothers and grandmothers. Exploring what this passing down might be, a modelling, or a genetic predisposition, perhaps nature or nurture, whatever the sense might be, can bring a sense of permission giving, an "I don't need to do it the way my mother did".

Any injunctions are possible. However, some seem more prevalent than others, such as Don't feel, Don't be you, Don't be important, Don't be safe, Don't achieve (as a parent). Particular driver behaviour is also seen in the maternal stages. Be Perfect is one of the most common drivers and can cause high, if not extreme, levels of perfectionism, paranoia and obsession – about the baby, the pregnancy, about health (baby's, partner's, mother's health) and high levels of catastrophising about death – that the baby will be stillborn, that the mother or infant (or both) will die in childbirth, or that something will occur to the partner, leaving them on their own to bring up the infant. Perfectionism and catastrophising bring the desire to control, and this often manifests as extreme control.

Many women try their utmost to be the best mothers they can but then feel a failure because they find aspects of parenting so difficult or out of their control. This can be a problem, particularly if the woman is used to being in a great deal of control, such as in the home or at work. Women in professions where control is paramount, such as the legal profession, banking or accountancy, can experience a heightened sense of failure when they realise their infant cannot be controlled in the way they had presumed would happen post birth. Some mums are absolutely obsessed with controlling their child's eating habits for fear of being told by their health visitor, friends or family that their infant is fat. This can cause them to restrict and monitor absolutely anything and everything that goes into their child's mouth, even stopping the child from participating in children's parties or going to tea with their friends due to high levels of fear of loss of control.

Breastfeeding can also be a problem. The push by medical professionals that "Breast is Best", although important, can be unhelpful and discouraging to some mothers. Those mums that find it difficult can experience a real sense of failure. It is equally distressing for those not producing enough for their starving infant. Not all women can breastfeed successfully, and some can keep persisting due to a sense that they will be considered a bad mum if they don't breastfeed their child. Yet, stress may also have a detrimental impact on milk production. Yes, breastfeeding is important for a newborn. Equally, it is not the be-all and end-all, and mothers are self-critical enough already without the medical profession and society increasing this and stigmatising them.

Some medical professionals also have a somewhat unfortunate habit of being perceived as judgemental. This can leave women feeling like a failure for reasons such as their infant is not thriving or because they are told they have put on too much weight during pregnancy. Weight monitoring, particularly commenting on weight gain, seems to be a recent trend in antenatal check-ups, particularly in the UK national health service. I can imagine it may have a lot to do with the increase in obesity in the UK. However, the line between helpful advice and fat shaming can be exceptionally narrow, and mums tell me how devastating it is to be told by a midwife that they are overweight.

The Be Strong driver can lead to a sense of being invisible and even to a sense of catastrophic thinking. However, there is a dichotomy here because women silence themselves, masking how they really feel, often showing racket feelings and behaviour (English, 1972) instead, and don't ask for help, so help cannot be forthcoming. This may be due to a perception of help not being available from a partner, family or friends, or medical professionals who might offer little treatment other than antidepressants. Women struggle on, feeling wretched, but not able to complain or do much other than just get on with it.

Having a Try Hard driver can lead to exhaustion, depletion of capacity and lack of energy. It is important to be mindful that there could be an underlying medical cause for these, such as iron deficiency, which can be debilitating and cause some women to feel almost unable to get themselves up and onto their feet. Exhaustion and a feeling of depletion are common. It is not okay to dismiss this as normal due to the sleep deprivation that comes with a newborn. Yes, there is sleep deprivation, but more than this, everyone has different energy levels. One mother may find it impossible to do much more than continuously breastfeed and watch Netflix and not much else; another may be quite able to head out to do their weekly shop with two other toddlers in tow, juggling newborn, shopping, toddler tantrums, school runs and anything else that comes her way.

Symbiosis between mother and infant is normal, natural and critically important. However, it can become difficult if the mother tips into obsession and becomes engulfing. This might be due to her own experience of abuse, neglect and trauma, giving her a heightened sensitivity to her children being impacted in this way. This can cause some parents not to allow their children to participate in sleepovers, to obsessively restrict the child from sugary products, or access to television, radio, computers and technology. None of these things, in themselves, are a problem. However, they can be useful discussion points if they seem overly restrictive or pathological. Discovering my client is still co-sleeping with their 11-year-old is a valuable topic of discussion, for example. However, I am mindful of bringing these into the dialogue in a way that is as natural as possible, being curious and open-minded rather than inflexible and rigid. It is useful to hold in mind different religious and cultural norms and keep them separate from the discussion. What may seem okay to me might not be so for my client, or vice versa. Offering space for my client to impart their normal for me to learn from can be eye-opening and helpful.

Other theoretical elements that are useful to note are passive behaviours (Schiff & Schiff, 1971) and discounting. Leaving aside the personal and professional quagmire that the Schiffs and their particular style of reparenting brought to TA, which I acknowledge brought untold harm to transactional analysis as a theoretical construct, particularly in the US, I find Cathexis theory (originally developed by Jacqui Schiff to treat psychosis and includes theories such as radical reparenting, redefining, discounting, frame of reference, symbiosis and passivity) helpful when working in the maternal. Due to the nature of parenting, it almost seems like passive behaviours and the discount matrix are unfolding in the therapy room before me. I am loathe to say that some parents are 're-parenting' themselves during the parenting process due to the risk of being shot down by those who would prefer to render this theory invisible or ostracise it completely. Yet, this is almost precisely what I see before me when a new parent, who may have had a very negative experience of being parented, chooses a very different way to parent their child. Is this script change (Berne, 1961)? Perhaps, for some, this is a helpful way of thinking about it. Our own children have the capacity to teach us a great deal about ourselves, and about those elements we did not have in our childhood: play, love, care, attachment, relational connection, regulation and the importance of permanence or object constancy. I find it useful to actively encourage new parents to learn from their infant.

Institutional and Systemic Racism within the Maternal System

I want to bring racism into the discussion about assessment and diagnosis because within the maternal system, particularly in the UK and the US, and almost certainly in other countries, there is most definitely institutional and systemic racism. I am not an expert in this area. However, the more there is an awareness about racism, and it is acknowledged, there is a possibility that it will begin to be addressed. That is my hope. I would very much like to be part of a culture that is truly accepting of and welcoming to anyone, regardless of who they are. Within the maternal, and particularly within the medical professions, this is not the case at all, and I find it unacceptable that this continues.

The most profound difficulties for Black and Mixed-race mothers I hear are that they feel invisible and dehumanised because when they ask for help, they are ignored, dismissed, or told that they do not feel pain. This is unacceptable and is clearly due to the myth, from slavery, that Black people do not feel pain. It is shocking that there are still reports of health inequity for Black and Mixed-race mothers (Snipe, 2022; Trawalter, 2022) and that research from Hoffman et al. (2016) showed that medical students in the US still believed that Black people felt less pain than White people. This causes Black and Mixed-race women to feel silenced and 'othered'.

In Chapter Two, I highlighted the very real lack of safety and security for Black and Mixed-race women when pregnant, giving birth and within the first-year post birth. In the UK, miscarriage is 40% higher in Black women than White women and economic deprivation seems to be behind higher incidences of stillbirth. To try to address this, there is a new governmental task force (the Maternal Disparities Taskforce) which hopes to tackle some of the disparities and inequalities in maternity care.

Intersectionality, wherever we are in the world, is complex and cannot be assumed or ignored within the therapy room. Being mindful of differences in cultural and religious traditions around childbirth is hugely important. Also, it is very dangerous to assume we know what a person's intersectionality is. For example, genetic disorders such as sickle cell anaemia can still be missed by medical staff even now when testing for this type of genetic condition is expected to be mandatory. It can be missed due to the assumption that the mother is of a specific ethnicity, when she may not be, yet is not asked directly, possibly due to fear in the professional of getting it wrong. Making no assumptions and speaking with clients with no bias or sense of shock is helpful but difficult and needs practice. I might perhaps not agree with a particular cultural tradition. For example, I am not Jewish or Muslim, so I do not have a sense of the importance of circumcision. Yet, I can understand how important this might be to explore, particularly with a couple where there is conflict around this practice, because, for one, it is hugely important, due to their religion and culture, yet for the other, it is an absolute boundary and a "no".

It is possible to explore and reflect on the rawness of information from bias, racism, and cultural and ethnic dissonance and be willing to somehow provide an empathic bridge, particularly if the therapist's knowledge and experience are not in alignment with their client's. For example, for some clients, my being White will be a hindrance, meaning that I cannot 'know' their experience of being othered. I cannot know how dehumanising it is to be invisible and unheard from the position of being Black. I absolutely agree with this, as there is no way I can know what this is like. I can, and have a duty to learn about my own racism and bias, to acknowledge it, explore it, and confront it, in whatever way I can.

Less Common Presentations

I want to briefly highlight a few presentations, for instance, tokophobia, hyperemesis gravidarum, infertility, ART, and stillbirth or neonatal death that women may bring with them into therapy. These are not necessarily unusual, but they may be unknown. The reason for this is that they are rarely spoken about, possibly a taboo subject for women and may bring fear of judgement and shame. Hyperemesis finally received some media coverage in the UK because Katherine, the Princess of Wales, experienced it during all three of her pregnancies.

Tokophobia

Tokophobia is a pathological and extreme fear of pregnancy and can lead to an avoidance of giving birth (Hofberg & Brockington, 2000). It can be so debilitating that women may abstain from sex entirely because their fear of becoming pregnant is so high. This intense phobia can stem from a number of things. There may have been something that happened in childhood, causing a distressing fear of needles, being sick, or fear of doctors and hospitals, which can severely impact a woman in her relationships, having a sex life, and any thoughts about having children. Some women are known to be unwilling to chance having sex at all. Others take precautions, using several methods of birth control at once. Sometimes the phobia is so great that even if the woman desperately wants a child, she won't contemplate going through with pregnancy and childbirth.

There are two types of tokophobia – primary and secondary. Primary is thought to stem from adolescence and occurs in those who have never been pregnant. Secondary tokophobia is due to a traumatic event that occurred either in pregnancy or during labour, such as stillbirth or birth trauma which then impacts any future thoughts of pregnancy or labour.

Tokophobia manifests itself in an intense fear of becoming or being pregnant. Unlike the majority of women who feel excitement at the prospect of being pregnant, women with tokophobia may feel no excitement at all and may instead feel intense terror and anxiety. If they fall pregnant, they may even consider termination. Causes can be childhood sexual abuse or rape, body dysmorphia or an intense fear of exposing the vagina or that health care providers might touch the vagina during childbirth. Tokophobia has been dismissed within health care settings. However, women who experience this pathological fear and who are then refused their choice of delivery may develop morbid fear and be at risk of requiring psychiatric care with any impending birth. It affects around 6–10% of pregnancies (Billert, 2007) and was shown to exist in higher levels of women due to the COVID-19 epidemic (Studzińska et al., 2022).

As with other types of phobia, I have found that tokophobia responds well to psychological treatment. I usually use a combination of relational TA and Eye Movement Desensitisation and Reprocessing (EMDR), which can be extremely effective in reducing the phobia aspect. I combine the two because I find this more powerful than using either on their own.

Hyperemesis Gravidarum

Hyperemesis gravidarum is extreme nausea and sickness in pregnancy which is often so debilitating that it requires hospitalisation so the woman can receive intravenous medication. Nausea and vomiting in early pregnancy are common and affect around 94% of all pregnancies. However, hyperemesis is a type of extreme sickness that only happens to around 3% of pregnant women and can last more than 20 weeks of the pregnancy. For some, it has such a detrimental impact on their food and fluid intake that it causes weight loss and severe dehydration, hence why hospital treatment may be needed.

The risk with hyperemesis is that a woman can go through childbirth seriously depleted, which can cause complications after birth, such as anaemia, depletion of energy, dizziness, confusion and disorientation. Support is important, particularly to encourage women to seek medical help, as they may feel so depleted that this might seem difficult. Help may come in the form of anti-sickness medication that a doctor can prescribe. Supporting the woman to be able to advocate for herself without feeling shame and stigma is also important. Many women will discount their experience of hyperemesis, yet it can lead to a miserable pregnancy that can feel never-ending. As hyperemesis is not being widely talked about, many women can feel isolated and alone, like they are the only person this has happened to.

Infertility

Coming to terms with infertility can be extremely difficult when, for some, they have desperately wanted to have children, often for many years. Infertility can be due to all manner of reasons, and it can put pressure on the strongest of partnerships. Pressure may come from experiencing the grief and loss from miscarriages, the need to go through numerous rounds of often quite expensive IVF, the invasive testing, and also a sense of anger towards the other if they are the infertile one. Infertility is often unspoken about and very much unwanted and can lead to unwelcome, overwhelming and extremely painful emotions.

Helping a couple who are experiencing infertility may highlight any disparities in the processing of grief. It is not at all uncommon for one person to seem to be at a different stage in their grief, leaving the other feeling a sense of disbelief, a "how could you be ok with this", or feeling misunderstood and alone. In these situations, I may suggest that the person who is struggling with their infertility continues in therapy alone on a long-term basis, as it can take time to fully explore the complex emotions that may surface, such as intense anger, rage and envy. It is also useful to explore what the couple want going forward. Some want help to come to terms with their infertility, deciding to stop trying and focusing on how they can live as a couple without resentment. Some may decide to try fostering or adoption. Some couples may choose artificial reproductive techniques to try and have the family they so desire, using donated eggs or sperm or finding a surrogate to carry the baby for them.

Artificial Reproductive Techniques

ART is the use of egg or sperm donors due to infertility. This can bring up many difficult decisions and considerations, particularly what this might mean for the couple, how they each feel about the donation, how it might be achieved and from whom. There may also be legal implications, which need to be explored fully. In some countries (the UK, for example), once a donor-conceived child reaches 18, they can apply to find the donor's identity and this may have a negative impact on the parents and bring tension between parents and child. There may be other implications, too, such as the donor having the right to withdraw consent for the embryo to be used for implantation. Couples, therefore, need to go into ART fully knowing what this means for them personally and legally.

There are many areas useful to explore when a couple choose ART. For example, if a donor is needed, would it be more advisable to use donors for both sperm and egg, so that neither parent feels at a disadvantage, or less connected with the infant? I have worked with couples where this has become a problem post-birth. In particular, if the woman is unable to become pregnant using her own egg and then uses a donor, yet the egg is fertilised using her partner's sperm, this can bring a sense of doubt in who is the 'mother', the woman who donates the egg or the woman who carries the infant. Having the ability to explore this prior to ART can be useful as many couples do not think about these implications.

There is also the possibility of going abroad for ART. Some couples may want to do this to circumvent some of the legal implications in their country of residence. However, it may be worth suggesting they explore any implications of this. When offering therapy for couples or clients with infertility issues, current knowledge of any legal implications and up-to-date research is useful.

Stillbirth and Neonatal Death

Stillbirth and neonatal death are extremely distressing to experience, and the parents may feel as if their lives have completely disintegrated. Stillbirth and neonatal death are terms used when a baby dies before or shortly after birth. There is no universal definition of when a fetus is considered stillborn or a miscarriage. Neonatal death is death within the first 28 days post birth. In the UK, stillbirth is after 24 weeks gestation, and in the US, it is after 20 weeks gestation. For the World Health Organization, babies who die after 28 weeks of pregnancy but before or during birth are considered stillborn. In the UK, around 13 families per day experience stillbirth or neonatal death (4,500 per annum). In Australia, this figure is about eight per day (6 stillborn, 2 neonatal deaths). It is uncommon, but it is not a rare occurrence; yet it can be utterly devastating, and simple daily activities can feel challenging and worthless after experiencing a stillbirth.

It is now more usual for parents to be given time to be with their baby and to create some memories after stillbirth or neonatal death. Midwifery services are much more supportive and understand just how distressing such a loss is, particularly as there are often no explanations for why the baby died. It can also bring extreme fear if a mother becomes pregnant again, and she can seem to be paranoid, quite understandably, as she will want cast-iron guarantees that this will not happen again and may be perceived as quite demanding of the obstetric team. Support groups for mothers can be beneficial, helping them to feel less alone in their grief, and offering a space to speak with other mums about their experiences. Fathers also benefit from support groups for stillbirth, even though many will try to hide their grief, or may be perceived to be grieving in a different way.

Neurodivergence

Neurodivergence or being neurodivergent includes minority neurotypes such as autism, attention-deficit hyperactive disorder (ADHD), dyslexia, dyscalculia, dysgraphia, dyspraxia, Tourette Syndrome, OCD, and epilepsy and there is also a huge range of diversity within each of these terms.

What is known is that women with neurodivergence can experience pregnancy and motherhood as complicated. For those with ADHD, routines can be challenging. For those who are autistic, they may prefer routine and order. If the mother has both, these can cause tensions, as her autism and ADHD may pull in opposite directions.

Autistic mothers and birth parents may have different experiences of pregnancy, birth and the postnatal period due to particular hypersensitivities and are at increased risk of pre-term birth due to higher levels of stress (Behrman & Butler, 2007). These sensory differences can make pregnancy and childbirth challenging (Ben-Sasson et al., 2009) due to hyper-sensitivity to sensory stimuli (touch – breastfeeding; sound – baby crying/noisy toys; interoception – internal feelings, pregnancy change, for example). They also may experience their emotions differently and find it difficult to express them, which can be diagnosed as something called alexithymia (Bird & Cook, 2013). These emotions can be overwhelming, painful, and distressing for the mother and cause her difficulties in adapting to her new role (Sundelin et al., 2018). Also, many parenting, communication and relationship expectations are based on normative assumptions which may not apply to autistic mothers.

Mothers who are neurodivergent often feel a more intense sense of shame, guilt and fear – very intense emotions which others may perceive as much more intense than is called for. This can cause neurodivergent mothers to feel inadequate as a parent, that they do not know what other mothers know. They may have an intense fear of asking for help, due to the shame of needing it in the first place. Having to rely on others because they feel they cannot cope as parents, because their sensitivity to emotion may feel overwhelming or so intense, can mean that they quickly feel emotionally exhausted, depleted and depressed.

Also, for mothers who find out they have a child with neurodivergence, if they consider themselves to be neurotypical, this can be distressing and bring with it guilt or concern that somehow they caused this to happen within the pregnancy. In particular, mothers who were ambivalent prior to and during pregnancy can experience extreme guilt if the child is then diagnosed with autism. It is important to offer the space for parents to really explore how they feel about their child's diagnosis, as they may find their own emotions difficult to deal with, and particularly shaming. For a more in-depth exploration of neurodivergence, please see my first book, *Motherhood and Mental Illness* (Haynes, 2022b), as I have a chapter on neurodivergence.

Gender Identity and Parenthood

There seems to be a myth, or perhaps an idea, that people who are transgender or who identify as non-binary will not be interested in parenthood. This is not correct at all. However, unsurprisingly, there is little known about the psychosocial impact on the family formation dilemmas of transgender and non-binary adults, mainly because there is not enough research. Research by Marinho et al. (2020) shows that a considerable number of those who are actively engaged in gender transition want to have children in the future and are balancing a desire for parenthood and desires for other life goals.

There is a conjoined challenge of gender and fertility because there may be a need for the use of artificial reproductive techniques. However, the search for a non-binary or gender-appropriate service, or one in which the need for flexibility in future planning centred on reproductive capacity can be difficult, if not impossible. There can also be a sense that "who I am" does not fit the cisgender system of fostering, adoption and fertility services.

Research has shown that about half of all transgender men (Wierckx et al., 2012) and transgender women (De Sutter et al., 2002) desire to have a genetically related child. And over one-third of transgender men said they would consider cryopreservation if these techniques were available, and over three-quarters of transgender women thought that egg and sperm freezing should be routinely offered before hormonal treatment (De Sutter et al., 2002).

At present, fertility preservation is not routinely offered to all transgender and non-binary people prior to undergoing gender-affirming hormonal treatments. In the US, fertility preservation is very expensive and is not routinely covered through medical insurance. In the UK, only a few centres offer a service for storing gamete tissue. Due to the age that people now present for gender surgery, this now presents an issue regarding fertility preservation (Barrett, 2022).

There is also the added complexity of issues faced by transgender and non-binary people who are living beyond cisnormativity, and who are trying to tread a difficult and interwoven course of considerations in their decision to become or not to become parents. There are challenges which are both medical and societal in nature. Transgender and non-binary people say they feel a sense of ignorance, discrimination and prejudice towards them and perceive this will continue with their parenting choices. There is also an absence of appropriate funding for any kind of fertility treatment, and many anticipate that there would be difficulties if they tried to adopt, due to their anticipation of not being approved as suitable (Tasker & Gato, 2020).

As therapists, our role may be to help them advocate and question the parenting opportunities for transgender and non-binary people and to assist them in asking about the possibilities of fertility preservation after any form of hormonal or surgical treatments.

Ethical Dilemmas

I want to highlight a few ethical dilemmas here to bring them into the open, as there are many gritty and troublesome dilemmas from pre-conception through to the post-birth period, many of which can cause tension in the therapist and the client. Although there is not space to speak about these fully, I want to name just a few here, and to offer some questions to consider.

Ethical dilemmas offer an opportunity to promote thinking and exploration as well as dialogue about cultural, religious, familial and political belief systems, all of which are alive and present in motherhood and parenthood. For example, if our client has been informed her infant will not survive until term due to serious medical complications and she is faced with a decision to terminate the infant due to medical reasons (TFMR) what is our role? How do we hold our own thoughts and views outside the therapy room and do no harm? What about working with a teenage client who is pregnant due to incest and rape, or a couple who continue to seek IVF after losing multiple embryos? These types of dilemmas can be fraught with different difficulties.

What about if we are working across borders and seeing a client in, for example, Romania, who is experiencing a dilemma because she wants to give birth naturally but has been told by her obstetrician that this is not possible and that she needs to be booked in for a Caesarean-section? Research is showing that there are now alarming rates of C-sections occurring in some countries – such as in Egypt, Bulgaria and Romania (Visser et al., 2018). There is also evidence from Johanson, Newburn and Macfarlane (2002) that even straightforward pregnancies are now often subject to routine interventions, with a concern that there is an over-medicalisation of childbirth in many countries throughout the world. It is likely that this over-medicalisation may continue as the male body has always been the norm in medical and scientific research – meaning that women's conditions are often missed altogether, misdiagnosed, or completely unresearched.

A small selection of questions to consider

How often do we think clearly about who we are as a person and who we might be as a parent?

Is there something wrong if I don't want children?

What will happen to me in old age if I don't have a child to support me?

How can I come to terms with never giving birth – will I hold regret?

How do we put our own bias aside when a client who is morbidly obese and so determined to have a child continues to pay for round after round of IVF treatment in a private fertility clinic to no avail?

What if the woman is pregnant and has intense doubts about going through with the pregnancy, but it is too late to have an abortion?

What do we do when a client is harming themselves yet is unable to see this as self-harm because their vision is clouded?

At what point do we help the client to grieve and tolerate their infertility?

Is it our role to help clients to understand that it is futile to continue to hope?

Whose choice is it to terminate a pregnancy?

What if the pregnancy was a mistake or was due to rape or sexual abuse?

What if the woman knows the abuser or he is a relation or family friend?

What if the woman does not want to involve the father and is determined not to tell them?

What about religious or cultural implications and dilemmas if termination is forbidden?

How do we support women who are deeply shamed about weight gain during pregnancy?

How can I help a woman who is blaming her baby for her birth trauma?

How do I feel about a woman giving birth to a baby and giving it up for adoption?

How do I support a woman who has experienced medical negligence, yet believes she is the one who was at fault?

Conclusion

In this chapter, I have highlighted the differences between assessment and diagnosis and listed some of the most common presentations that may be seen. I have also sought to encourage reflection on ethical dilemmas, working with gender identity and parenthood, infertility, artificial reproductive techniques and neurodivergence and some of the unspoken but not uncommon presentations such as tokophobia and hyperemesis gravidarum. This chapter is not exhaustive. What I hope can be taken from it is the vastness of this type of work and the multitude of diverse presentations which can and will crop up in the therapy room.

4

HEALING THROUGH RELATIONSHIP
Relational TA

I am a relational transactional analyst. I work with and through the relationship with my maternal clients because this is effective, valuable and rewarding. I could not conceive of working any other way when I am often confronting the most profound and unpredictable relational disturbances. Such disturbances can often also evoke agitation in the parental protocol. The birth of a baby has the capacity to awaken the earliest unconscious processes. The mother can be taken to the extremes of emotion, with an intensity that can be utterly terrifying, and to places of desperation, despair, envy, rage, love and grief.

Relationship sits at the core of the maternal, and relationship disturbances sit at the core of maternal mental illness. At all times, my focus is on a dual relationship – mother with fetus/infant; parent with child; not-yet parent with unborn infant. I use my curiosity and creativity to focus on what I consider to be the most fundamental elements in my work: safety and security, connection, attachment, bonding and disturbance, working within the transferential domain. These elements help my client and me to unpick their relationship difficulties with the aim and hope of enhancing their ability to engage, attach, connect and bond with themselves, with important others and with their baby in the present moment and going forward. Human relationality is also fundamentally encoded in our DNA due to our inability to survive without others. I expand on this encoding in Chapter 5.

I use a broad range of TA theories as I find TA diverse and rich, much as my clients are also diverse and rich. This offers me a spectrum of possibilities and choice of interpretation. This diversity is useful, as a theory may help clarify my understanding of one mother, but may not fit at all with another. I also acknowledge that my way of relational working is uniquely mine and may not be remotely the same as other TA therapists.

Humans are relational beings from conception and continue in relationships with others throughout their lives. Even before conception, some parents fantasise about their possible future infants and show aspects of being in a relationship with that fantasy infant. More than this, humans are also always interconnected to, influenced by and in relationship with their environment. These relationships – to others and the environment – influence how each

DOI: 10.4324/9781003365822-4

human perceives the quality of their life and their frame of reference, and give meaning to their everyday human being. It is this fundamental need for and impact of these relationships, encoded within human DNA, that speaks to me of the importance of working in this way with my maternal clients.

When I use the word environment, I am attempting to encapsulate any surroundings or conditions humans live in, past, present and future. The word environment might mean many things: the womb in which the fetus is growing; the familial environment; the physical (human-built) surroundings; the emotional and psychological environment; nature and the natural environment (non-human-made); it will also include those negative unsafe environments full of toxicity, fear and insecurity. Connection to and with our environment, particularly nature (both psychologically and physically), has many influences on our health and well-being (Barragan-Jason et al., 2023) and is bi-directional.

For me, relational psychotherapy hinges on *self with other*, in precisely the same way that the mother/infant dyad hinges on *self with mother*. My focus is primarily on the mother's relational connections, or their lack, and the influence her historical dynamics have on these connections in the present moment. It is essential to acknowledge that *self with other* includes my own sense of myself with the other and my own historical dynamics. I need to pay close attention to my sense of self because if it is being impacted by severe stress or by other factors, or it is lacking in some way; my self-relationship may impact the work with my maternal client, and would almost certainly be a re-enactment of past relational disturbances. Thus, ongoing depth therapy is necessary, as is plentiful good supervision, with those capable of critiquing my thinking and behaviour.

From the first exchange, how the client interacts with me offers me a sense of my client's experiences of their relationships and, in particular, those very first relational dynamics. This helps me build a picture of possible survival strategies and defences a person may have had to use to remain in a relationship and will play a vital part in working with the mother/infant relationship. More than this, it gives me clues about how we might be together and what my client may want and need in therapy. However, it is vital not to make assumptions or for me to think I know what is going on. I won't.

Relational Psychotherapy

The central tenet of relational psychotherapy is healing through relational connection, the relationship between self and other. Those who advocate this type of psychotherapy do not necessarily believe an individual holds the sole power to fix themselves and is totally responsible for their own happiness. Instead, relational psychotherapy, as I conceive it, changes the focus towards togetherness, acknowledging that a stable, healthy, strong connection can give a person power and agency, and promote physis to live the life they want to. Similarly, these are aspects that are vitally important to promote healthy functioning from infancy.

Hargaden and Schwartz (2007) identify several key elements in relational psychotherapy which Tudor (2014) listed as:

- The centrality of the relationship
- Therapy as a two-way street involving a bi-directional process
- The vulnerability of both therapist and client is involved
- Countertransference is used not merely as information but in thoughtful disclosure and collaborative dialogue
- The co-construction and multiplicity of meaning.

(Hargaden & Schwartz, 2007, p. 4)

The belief is that change occurs through the relational dyad because the client and therapist are interacting together and impacting each other and can co-construct meaning about this interactional, impactful process, in which the past will be influencing and colouring the present moment. Again, there are similarities with this and the mother/infant dyad. Change, however, does not occur if the therapist and/or client are unwilling to be impacted (altered in some way) by the other and by the process. Thus, it is a bi-directional process. Historical negative repetitive relational patterns will occur within therapy, and these unconscious processes have the power to thwart the present moment relating, usually resulting in mistakes and splits (enactments). These mistakes (often called ruptures) offer the possibility to inform the present therapeutic relationship and are an opportunity to gain an understanding of the client's struggles.

The Need for a More Individualised Treatment

The movement towards a more relational approach to psychotherapy has been ongoing for the last 30 or so years and originated from a perceived need to counter goal-oriented, more solution-focused protocols, or 'one-size-fits-all' styles of psychotherapy that seemed to be focused on the therapist's (or mental health service's) need rather than the client's. These protocols can place a barrier between therapist and client, stopping the therapist being altered in any way, shape or form by the client. This type of treatment is not for me, as I believe those with perinatal mental illness want to be heard, acknowledged and witnessed in their distress. I do not believe a manualised system will offer the same possibilities for maternal clients to grow psychologically, in terms of both their ability to tolerate their maternal distress and in their reflective capacity as a mother.

Within the perinatal field, in national health services worldwide, protocols (a detailed plan of treatment procedure on a session-by-session basis) or routine competency frameworks may mean greater access to help and are easier and cheaper to provide. However, the efficacy of treatment protocols for those women receiving this treatment may be questionable, as trying to shoehorn maternal clients into a protocol does not necessarily work as well as it might. As yet, research rarely asks perinatal women to rate their treatment from medical services. In my small research study (Haynes, 2019) and from my work over the last decade, most of my clients have said they came to therapy in private practice due to their dissatisfaction with either the lack of provision of perinatal services, or because that provision was not satisfactory. In the very few perinatal mental health services existing in the UK, some basic routine measures are now being used. Whether the data is analysed and used is unclear, although there does not seem to be anything published yet (late 2023). As this book is intended for psychotherapists in private practice, it aims to suggest a more tailored, flexible, individualized style of therapy to offer the greatest chance for perinatal clients to gain long-term benefits.

Over the last 30 years, a growing number of psychotherapists recognized their clients were coming with ever more complex presentations that traditional theory could not explain nor treat adequately and that a more flexible approach might be helpful. During the time I have worked in the maternal field, I have also recognized the increases in complexity of presentation. At the same time, advancements in science, neurobiology, and human development took off, and research was able to offer tangible explanations about brain functionality and the human psyche. Neuroscience is now advancing at speed, as is the scientific understanding of the way in which cortisol, epinephrine and adrenaline impact human emotion and the repercussions of these. It is now even possible to use functional MRI scanning to see the unborn fetus and to gain important information about development in the womb. This new knowledge has been combined with a recognition of the need for a more biopsychosocial approach to mental health.

Relational psychotherapy seeks to focus on the client's expertise in themselves and their processes, putting the client in the position of knowing. This would incorporate my belief in and focus on the specificity of each of my maternal clients' perinatal experiences. Within the perinatal sphere, research shows that the specificity of treatment and its relevance to the woman's experience is an important factor in the success of that treatment (O'Mahen et al., 2015). Kwan, Dimidjian and Rizvi (2010), in their research on treatment for depression, also show that people who received their treatment of choice were more likely to begin and then remain in treatment. As there is evidence to show high levels of attrition or non-completion of treatment (Austin et al., 2008; Meager & Milgrom, 1996) within perinatal mental illness, providing a style of treatment that focuses on the client's particular difficulties and places them as the expert seems to be common sense. Unfortunately, this is at odds with the medical model of illness promoted by most national health services and within the medical professions.

Yet, no two women will ever have experienced the same conception, pregnancy or birth experience, nor require the same process in therapy. There may be similarities in client experiences, and this can be a slippery slope into assuming that we (therapists, medical professionals) know what the client's experience is and how it should be 'fixed'. We don't know. Assumption may also be quite a dangerous position for a therapist, although it is easy to find oneself in it. I prefer to attempt to honour the client's unique experience and allow the sessions to be flexible enough to incorporate this individuality. I use the word 'attempt' purposefully. Dependent upon the strength and pull of unconscious processes, this does not necessarily come easily.

Strengthening the Therapeutic Alliance

Relational psychotherapy hinges on the therapeutic alliance, one of the core processes. Perinatal psychotherapy calls for an acute awareness of the thera-peutic alliance, because it will be rich with information on the woman's alli-ance with her own mother. For the therapeutic alliance to be strong enough to withstand the ups and downs and inevitable mistakes or ruptures within the work, there is an acknowledgement of the need for the therapist to be part of the process with their client rather than being separate from it. This is rooted in a recognition that sitting in a position of observing the relationship from a distance (being apart from the process) is not the same as being in it and may not offer the client the best opportunity for relational change.

In fact, if I was to be apart from the process rather than in it, this may again be a re-enactment of an early experience in childhood of an observing yet distant or withdrawn mother. This might be a mother who is abandoning her infant by watching but not attending to her infant's distress. Research by Lyons-Ruth (Lyons-Ruth & Yarger, 2022) shows just how damaging this type of distancing can be for an infant, which she believes may be the key to the foundational processes of borderline personality disorder. This type of mother is there (in the room) yet not connected and attending to the infant when that infant reaches out for connection. This type of mother leaves that infant alone in its own distress, which is utterly confusing for the infant, with its mother close by yet inattentive. Lyons-Ruth shows just how damaging this withdrawn behaviour can be. Indeed, many of my maternal clients have told me this expe-rience is like having a wall of glass between themselves and their mother, which they recognise because this behaviour continued and may still continue in the present moment. They can see their mother, but not yet touch or reach her. Their crying out enters an echo chamber of nothingness, leading to despair.

The bi-directionality of relational psychotherapy is ongoing, with the therapist focusing on moment-by-moment attunement, helping to keep the process client-focused. This parallels the need between mother and infant. Although, in both cases (psychotherapy and mother/infant connection) moment-by-moment attunement is impossible and not even useful as it is a fantasy position. Yet, much like with parenting, it is this repetitive, ongo-ing attempt for connection and attunement within the relationship, that is reparative. There needs to be a level of tolerance within the therapist, much like there is tolerance within the mother to sustain her through the repetitive nature of this need to be in attunement. What is useful is for it to be good enough. Good enough is what is good enough for the client, for the relationship, and for the connection to continue.

Relational psychotherapy offers the maternal client the opportunity to explore and discover such questions as "Who am I in relationship to another?", "How do I value myself, and how does this impact how others value me?" This is due to the belief that insight alone is not enough and that change comes from acquiring new, positive patterns of relationships with self and others. The shift towards a more relational approach came from the synthesis of different theories and has its roots within an integrative approach: incorporating British object relations theory and American interpersonal psychoanalytic thinking, existential thinking, feminist and postmodern thinking, and self-psychology.

Relational Transactional Analysis

Relational TA is not simply about interpretation or illustration. It is about forming a new relationship experience through connection and interaction, with the hope of opening up possibilities to change. For many of the parents I see, their relationship with their own mother and/or father is often difficult, and this can cause them to struggle with their relationship to their infant. The infant may be much wanted, yet once here, the mother may feel inept, overwhelmed, fearful and clueless. Whatever she is feeling, this is information.

In the here and now, my client and I are relating together, both experiencing the relationship, both hearing stories from the past that impact our present moment relating. Both of us are actively co-creating new meaning, new stories and new interactions. This type of psychotherapy requires us both to be active participants and, therefore, vulnerable to being shaped and changed by this process and by the enactments that will happen. I need to be willing to feel, acknowledge, work with and sometimes disclose my countertransference for the benefit of my client (not for my benefit). There is no preconception or agenda, which makes it difficult to achieve. It is not easy for the client either, as they require a commitment to stay in therapy, through all the repetitions of past dysfunctional relational patterns, which can be acutely painful to re-experience. However, within this repetition process, with time, dedication and empathy, something different and healing can slowly emerge.

Storytelling, narration and accounting for the multiplicity of meaning around these repeating patterns are an important part of the process. I notice how these stories begin to change over time, and I use this glimpse of the change process happening, which I feed back to my client. It is helpful to offer women a sense of change. Often, they do not notice it in themselves, so being able to notice their growth can be validating for them. Yes, it requires a type of loyalty from both therapist and client, a staying with and toleration of the process because for many with relational trauma, the 'other' (mother) did not stay – they walked away and abandoned the relationship. Fear of the inevitability of abandonment and neglect can override the client before any form of psychological repair can happen, which is why the ability to really reflect on our own process and also remain deeply empathic to the client's story, yet always retain a subjective sense of self, is so important.

I believe perinatal clients, perhaps much more than other clients, seem to require more of the therapist. The only way I have found to provide the 'more' has been through relational work. I wonder whether this is because of the nature of the work in the parental dyad, living and breathing those primary relationships, the positive symbiosis and enmeshment our clients have with their infants (unborn as well as born) who are trying to understand and care for their tiny infants in the best way they can. Certainly, this work brings a particular rawness in experience, working on the cusp of life and death (IVF, ART, infertility, TFMR, miscarriage, stillbirth, sudden infant death, terminal illness in an infant or child, for example). But more than this, it is the hope and expectation that any parent is filled with, and the disappointments and heartbreaks that occur with pregnancy, birth and parenting. Yes, all psychotherapists walk this path with their clients. However, I would argue that perinatal work requires something particular of a therapist and is not for everyone. Much like being a parent, it is filled with extreme highs and lows; it can be long term and requires capacity for patience and tolerance, much in the same way as parenting does, and an acceptance that shit really does happen in life and that fantasies are utterly unhelpful, yet absolutely inevitable. I also freely acknowledge that I am biased and that my passion for and bias towards my work influences the way I feel about it.

Conception, pregnancy and birth are suffused with strong transferential processes, and the lack of positive experience in being parented may bring a strong urge or need to do things differently with our own child(ren). It can also bring strong yet heavily defended fear that it might not be different, and that the same mistakes will be made, with a sense of inevitable failure in parenting. This 'push/pull' process can evoke fear and anxiety, is often intense and may come from a lack of safety and security in the earliest relationships, in which the client has been let down and damaged by their caregiver.

The provision of safety and security, therefore, becomes one of the most fundamental aspects in my maternal work, and this includes for me too. Without safety and security, the client may find engaging in therapy in the way needed to build a strong therapeutic alliance difficult, or even impossible. Safety and security permeate many different layers of relationship, and at the root, are the key to the therapeutic relationship. A parent who does not feel safe enough, or equally a mother who finds trust an impossible concept, may defend against therapy, finding fault in me or in the type of therapy I do, or simply decide it is not for them and walk away suddenly. Within my thinking, I treat trust as separate from safety and security. A client may never 'trust', and yet I can still offer them a safe enough space to feel secure enough to be in a relationship with me.

Some of my clients say they will never trust anyone, due to their extremely difficult historic relational struggles, most often with their mother or father, but sometimes with grandparents, aunts or uncles; the client encoded in such a way that the difficulties in forming an alliance are an inevitable part of life. Perhaps the client finds it difficult to share their innermost secrets, instead resorting to people pleasing, or shutting down communication through acting out in some way (becoming angry perhaps, or extremely emotional); perhaps they begin to play psychological games or show any number of behaviours not conducive to engagement or change. The difficulty of this inevitability of relational failure, is that it becomes transgenerational, handed down to the next generation. A struggle in forming relationships may also transcribe into a difficulty in the client bonding with their unborn child and disruptions with the attachment and bonding process post birth. Chapter 5 on Protocol expands my thinking and deepens this theory.

Relational Connection in Short- and Long-term Work

The areas of connection I am most interested in are attunement, attachment, bonding, connection, the transferential domain, and the intersubjective space between myself and my client. It is the connection between us that informs our work together, and I use our relationship for mutual understanding, facilitation and with the hope of moving the client towards a healing process. Without a strong, interpersonal relationship, something that takes time to build together, I find the change process can stall or falter.

However, due to what they might be coming with, some maternal clients may only need holding, interpretation and illustration. This does not mean therapy is not successful. There are many clients who have no need to prolong their therapy. An example of short-term relational work might be with a woman who is struggling in pregnancy, having lost a baby previously through stillbirth. This client may need a holding environment during her pregnancy to cope with her heightened anxiety and fear around another possible stillbirth. In this case, I would still deem the work as relational, as I would want to build a level of connection that can help the woman trust me enough so she can speak about her fears with no sense of judgement or fear of being labelled. This type of client work may never move out of holding. Yet, if she does not trust me enough, it is unlikely that her anxiety will lessen. Once her baby is safely born, an ending can often come quickly.

At the other end of the spectrum, there are many maternal clients who, even in relatively short-term work, can dive more deeply than they might have imagined. Working relationally is possible both in the long and short term, although the work is different. Depending on the issue the client is bringing, if it is a particular struggle with, for example, phobia (giving birth, being sick during pregnancy, needle-phobia), then I find short-term work, using elements such as Eye Movement Desensitisation and Reprocessing (EMDR) combined with relational psychotherapy can work well, as I stated in Chapter 3.

Intersubjectivity

Within the first phase of my relational work, there is always a gap between myself and my client, which is filled with the unknown. This is not too dissimilar to a mother and her newborn infant finding themselves with a sense of knowing, yet equally, it is an unknowing knowing. It takes time for mother and infant to get to know each other and for the mother to begin to understand what her infant wants and needs, and how this might or might not be fulfilled. This process can be filled with rupture or disconnection; the mother may feel as if she is getting it wrong, is assuming too much, or equally, she might feel at a loss of how to proceed. With some clients, particularly those who experienced severe developmental trauma, it can be uncanny how similar processes occur within the therapeutic dyad, the enactment leaving the client feeling unheard and the therapist feeling at a loss to 'know' what the client needs. It is clear that 'something' is needed. I am loathe to call this 'repair' (Safran et al., 2011), which seems to be the process advocated by some within relational transactional analysis. I prefer to use the word response, because it is the way in which this response is given that can be so hugely valuable, and the very fact that a response has been given, particularly for those clients who experienced neglect or abandonment. This is very similar to the importance of the response of the parent from an infant of around six months of age. This response becomes fundamental to the infant and how the infant begins to comprehend their parental caregivers. I believe it is this process of response that can be 'transformational' although I find this word problematic too, as calling it this runs the risk of discounting a process that has the capacity to be hugely difficult and painful, and which requires so much of both therapist and client. Also, not handled well, this process can seriously damage the client. Response is a word I also use in Chapter 6 when I talk about the mother/infant dyad and the importance of the need/response cycle.

The process of inevitable failure on the part of the therapist and the possibility of stepping into the void of the relational rupture and filling it with something that is responsive (acknowledgement, shock, apology, curiosity, for example) helps to close the intersubjective gap. Equally, the client can begin to understand that the therapist is indeed human and makes mistakes, as all humans do. Perhaps, also, these mistakes in therapy can have a different flavour about them than in the client's childhood, as they are usually not malicious, intentional or neglectful, even if this might be how the client experiences them. Hopefully, there is a willingness in the therapist to acknowledge the impact such mistakes may have on their client.

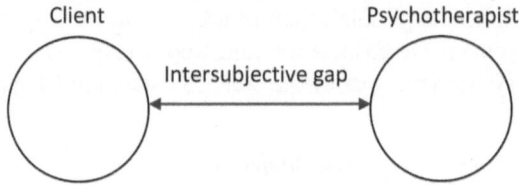

Figure 4.1 The First Phase of Relational Work: the Intersubjective Gap

This process is not dissimilar from the process of child development, which begins to be built from birth. Mothers fail their infants as they cannot always be there at every single moment. The child needs to learn to navigate this and to find ways to tolerate brief absences from their mother/caregiver. This is the beginning of the infant building a normal and needed capacity to self-soothe and entertain themselves for short periods of time. It is a natural and normal phase of a child developing executive function and self-regulation (for more in-depth theory about this, please see Key Concepts from the Centre on the Developing Child, n.d.). For a child who has good enough parenting, this is a natural developmental process. Yet, for a child with abusive or neglectful experiences of being parented, this process can be disrupted and may not happen at all.

In terms of the therapist/client relationship, the therapist will inevitably fail their client somehow. The client's response to these ruptures can give the therapist valuable insight into the deep relational processes at work. If the work is with a maternal client with developmental trauma, the success or failure of the work may depend on these times of rupture and how the therapist responds to them.

At the beginning of perinatal therapy, there is a large intersubjective gap (see Figure 4.1 above). Over time and getting to know one another, informed by the here and now responses and the back-there-and-then experiences, and with a good enough relational connection, the therapeutic alliance will begin to build, as shown in Figure 4.2, the horizontal arrows depicting movement towards one another.

With time, connection and commitment, client and therapist begin to move towards one another, forming a relationship in which the intersubjective

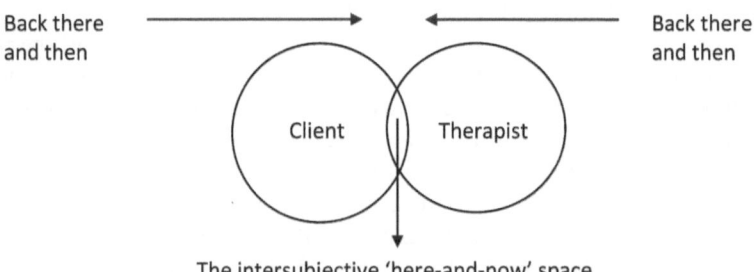

Figure 4.2 The 'Good Enough' Relationship

space can begin to form and be used. This is a space in which both therapist and client can begin to understand the bi-direction of the relationship, in which each impacts the other, co-creating the intersubjective space.

This is a simplistic explanation of what is a complex and often difficult process. However, there is no space to elaborate on this process more fully within this chapter. Also, it might sound as if I am saying that, in perinatal work, we need to fill the place of the good enough mother. This is not what I am saying at all. There are many parallels between relational therapy and mothering, and there is a real need to tread carefully and not get sucked into the deep, bottomless yearning for the 'perfect mother', and all that this negative, symbiotic dyad would become. This is why I caution the need for good, challenging supervision in which the work is critiqued.

Working relationally within the perinatal field can be difficult and is not for the faint-hearted. It is also possible, as a therapist, to find oneself in deep water very quickly through the inevitability of enactments, which occur out of awareness and seem to be impossible to stop. Once they have occurred, for therapy to continue and not falter, something needs to change.

I believe it is my role to step into the void of the enactment – to respond in a way that acknowledges my empathic failure because I will have missed something, some message from my client. It would be far too easy to project the misattunement back onto the client – "she played a game with me", "he was angry with me for abandoning him during my vacation". It is much more difficult, but necessary, to accept that the misattunement was almost certainly mine.

Yet, it is these misattunements, these relational 'failures' that offer so much more understanding of what is often deeply unconscious. This is much like Cornell and Bonds-White's (2001) comment: "for Bollas, as for Winnicott, empathic failure, rather than inevitably creating or recreating a narcissistic wound, can offer creative space and opportunity" (p. 79). The 'something' that is the response that needs to happen might be slowing the therapeutic process down perhaps, taking a step back from it, acknowledging to our client the pain and impact, allowing light and air into the process as a way towards understanding the essence of what happened. Enactments have the capacity to be deeply painful and shocking to both therapist and client, and hold such significance about the relational process, on a historical level and in the present moment. Supervision is a critical part of relational work and bringing the failures within the therapeutic process can often be enlightening, shaming and impactful. Equally, I would argue that supervision is not enough. We need to explore our part of the enactment in our own therapy if we hope ever to understand what sits beneath it.

Conclusion

Relational psychotherapy does not work for all maternal clients and may even be unnecessary or unfruitful for some. Some therapists baulk at it and find working in the transferential domain to be deeply disturbing and prefer to use manuals, instruments, measurements and protocols as a way of feeling safe in their work. It can be a struggle to remain open to the vicissitudes in the work, particularly if the client feels quite persecutory. The work can often feel messy, sticky, distressing and difficult. Thus working through a relational lens requires scrutiny and continuous critique, both internally through self-reflection (highlighting my own actions and responses) and externally, using supervision to question my actions and responses and therapy to truly understand why this happened in the first place. Only in this way can I hope to keep as firm a boundary as possible around my self, in order to focus on the client and place their needs foremost in the work.

Without strong boundaries, there is a real danger of enmeshment and symbiosis when working relationally with perinatal clients. Those who experienced difficult primary relationships, developmentally, can yearn for enmeshment, for a positive symbiosis that they may never have experienced, and this we know as introjective transference (Kohut, 1971) – the narcissistic transferences of mirroring, idealizing and twinship. Clients with developmental trauma (trauma from conception through to their earliest years) may unknowingly (and sometimes in awareness) evoke a strong pull, through these transferential processes, for the therapist to offer themselves up to merging with them. Kohut believed the task of therapy was to offer empathic attunement as a reparative experience. Offering empathy and attunement in this way could be viewed in TA theory as offering a new experience of a parental figure. Yet, there is also a strong possibility of idolisation and idealisation from clients with developmental trauma, which can be seductive to a therapist, particularly one with a combination of Be Perfect and Please Others drivers – hence, why self-care needs to be a crucial part of perinatal TA psychotherapy.

Another limitation of this type of work is around the possibility for therapist burnout. The possibility of burnout and the need for self-care are so important within relational psychotherapy that I have placed them in their own chapter (Chapter 12) with complex presentations. The perinatal, in particular, can be exacting on a therapist and there is a real need to focus on self-care and to take regular breaks in this work.

Finally, I do believe there is a limitation on how relational TA can be taught. We can speak of it theoretically. However, experientially, this type of psychotherapy is difficult to teach to students. It takes time and commitment to really understand the depth of relational work. Students may want to work in this way, but I find it difficult to explain adequately enough for them to comprehend the long-term commitment and requirements this type of therapy requires of the therapist, so that they can enter into this work fully understanding what it truly is.

5

EXPLORING THE DIALECTICS OF SURVIVAL AND POTENTIAL

Protocol

Written in collaboration with Ronen Stilman

Let's begin by exploring and expanding the TA term 'protocol' and why it is so relevant within maternal mental health. We[1] want to highlight our theory of protocol and the significance of it beginning to develop much earlier than birth. How is this tied to the human brain's development, particularly around safety and danger, which we believe forms a critical part of protocol? Before we explore protocol, let us explain what is meant by this term. Eric Berne first wrote about protocol in 1961 and used it to describe the feelings held within the body as, what he called, an unconscious primal 'image' about those experiences of others within our earliest years of life, from birth to around two or three years of age, that made a significant impression on us. It is important to start by saying that these feelings are not only pathological.

Protocol impacts us as we grow and evolve. We believe this impacts both positively and negatively three elements that are crucial: physis (the growth force); potential (that all humans are born with); and intuition, and these three elements form the difference between surviving and thriving. What if our protocol, our response to danger and our relational being is encoded to thwart our ability to thrive, our potential? What happens if our intuition is encoded in a way, due to our experiences in utero, that is not helpful to us? How does this shape us as we grow and evolve?

Protocol shapes all these important aspects – physis, potential, intuition, and is full of possibility – yet it can also be limiting. Within this chapter, we will explore our thinking around transgenerational protocol and how these might influence our script decisions, intuition and protocol. Finally, we would like to show the depth and breadth of nonconscious processes. We use, in particular, Cornell and Landaiche's (2008) concept of nonconscious processes "more than just a place in the mind ... an active, interpersonal dynamic that is central to human relations work" (p. 202). We also integrate Pierini's (2008) inclusion of implicit as well as out-of-awareness processes, from 'back there and then' as well as from 'here and now', any of which may be formed in utero. This transferential domain (for example, the body,

DOI: 10.4324/9781003365822-5

intuition and primal images) is essential in facilitating understanding of our client's nonconscious processes.

How is protocol important for motherhood, and why is it in the first few chapters on working with maternal mental illness using transactional analysis? Protocol is extremely relevant within the maternal due to the timespan in which it is formed in the fetus/infant – from conception to around two years of age – precisely when women can experience mental disturbance and distress. The maternal is absolutely critical in the formation of protocol, as it is often the mother who shapes the limiting and enabling factors of protocol, the encoded responses to safety and danger and the relational patterns and attachment process, and these, in turn, shape our future. These are the foundation of the frame of our potential, our possibility and can limit or thwart physis. We believe protocol is formed as part of the need for newborns to have the capacity to be both adaptive and self-regulatory in order to "cope with the highly diverse environment and various kinds of stimulation" (Lang et al., 2020, p. 837). The time frame in which protocol is formed is critical, yet it is often discounted and undermined socially, politically and economically. As already stated earlier in this book, the system, particularly in the Western world, is very good at blaming the mother but is very bad at supporting her when she most needs it. Within psychotherapy, there has also been a long-lived and continuous theme that the problem lies within the 'mother'. We will challenge this, both within psychotherapy and within society.

Our theory of protocol also supports our political thinking that there is a critical need for a paradigm shift in the way motherhood and maternal mental illness are framed: from one of individual blame and a significant systemic lack of care to a more encompassing understanding of the critical need for and provision of support during motherhood. Mothers are the containers of the future of humanity – the very essence of human potential and human survival. Surely, they warrant our greatest support.

It feels pertinent to include an in-depth exploration of protocol at the beginning of this book, as protocol of the fetus/infant and perhaps the mother too, may be impacted, stirred and disturbed by maternal mental illness and/or psychotherapy. Protocol can also be impacted by systemic factors – family, relationships, social unrest, war, migration, or ecological events, such as drought and famine for example. As Bollas eloquently puts it: "it is perhaps more accurate to see the mother – rather like a newspaper – simply conveys the news. The stories come from many sources" (2021, p. 2).

Protocol lays a psychological/emotional foundation for human being for the entirety of life and impacts humans, positively or negatively, whether they realise it or not, particularly if the person's earliest experiences were of neglect or harm. We believe protocol begins to be formed earlier than other TA theorists have stated, prior to birth, in utero. Indeed, it is possible that parts of our protocol may even be formed through a transgenerational process, which we would call transgenerational protocol, held at a cellular level perhaps, although whether this would be a part of our DNA is not known as yet.

Protocol may be viewed as what Cornell refers to as "both pre-ego and sub-ego, that is, preceding the developmental capacities for ego organization and underlying the functions of the ego throughout the course of life" (2008b, p. 143). We believe that one of the primary parts of protocol, and encoded within it, is our encoded response to safety and danger. Humans appear to be encoded to respond to safety and danger before everything else, possibly because without this, the human species simply would not survive. Our autonomic nervous system and our ability to respond to danger through the use of our senses is one of the first elements that develops in utero. These two elements, our threat response and our senses, develop together, almost certainly due to the need to instinctively 'pick up' the threat signal via our senses and respond without thinking. This links to transgenerational protocol and 'maternal effects'. If it is important for 'us' (our family, our community, our race, our village, etc.) to respond to a particular threat (the impact of slavery, persecution, war, famine, natural disaster perhaps ...), we believe that these experiences and knowledge are then held on a 'cellular' basis and passed down the generations through what we call transgenerational protocol, in order that future generations can adapt more quickly to survive within that environment. This handing down is likely to come through the maternal line due to maternal effects (Wolf & Wade, 2009) although we do not know this for sure. Not only this, protocol also encodes our relational patterns, and this is linked to safety and danger. We cannot survive without others, so it makes sense that a fetus/infant will need to expedite their relationships from the earliest possible moment. Apprey offers an expansion of this when talking of his theory of "transgenerational haunting", which he describes as an "alive" process that is powerful and phenomenological, a "possession", "**an ancestor who has returned and possesses an other body**" (2019, p. 340, original emphasis).

Protocol can be both vitalising and inhibiting, offering a limiting and potential state, dependent upon how it manifests in the given environment. The theory of protocol has the possibility of linking TA to other theories such as Polyvagal theory, trauma theory and attachment theory. We are building upon and extending some of Cornell's theory, particularly from his recent book *At the Interface of Transactional Analysis, Psychoanalysis and Body Psychotherapy* (2019). However, we believe we are bringing new developments to protocol by locating it as an encoded, developed and inherited response to safety and danger as well as to relationship forming. We believe that the way in which humans face safety and danger is shaped within protocol, which affects the capacity of their physis to materialise, which in turn impacts the potential they were born with. Is this the edge, the difference between survival and thriving?

All humans are born into and evolve within an environment crucial to their health and well-being. As such, we believe protocol is formed within familial environments, in an inter-relational process (Haynes, 2022b), something which will be explored in Chapter 13 of this book. We do not know categorically whether protocol can be formed in isolation, i.e. without 'others', but we don't believe that to be the case. Humans, particularly in their formative years, do not tend to survive alone. Their families, tribes or alternative group formations which provide aspects of 'family' will have a system of cohesion that holds them together; for example, attachment, intersubjectivity, culture and ideology. Such systems of cohesion will manifest in caring and supporting ways as well as in harmful and limiting ways, such as through abuse, slavery or co-dependency.

Protocol, as it is a foundational aspect of human development, warrants more discussion and research within TA theory, as the focus has been more firmly towards later stages of script development. Research is able to show how the gestational environment and the experiences of a fetus during conception and gestation can impact the fetus physically, socially, emotionally and cognitively for its entire lifetime (Weinstein, 2016). Protocol is formed in the exact same time frame that maternal mental illness normally occurs, and we believe the two impact each other. Thus, a thorough understanding of protocol and its role in life, any future decision-making and human 'becoming' is important.

The medical system cannot continue only to treat the individual, as acknowledgement is needed that the system the individual is conceived and evolves within is part of the problem. A systemic view would argue that maternal mental illness is a manifestation of disturbance in the familial system (Stilman, 2009). As the metaphor of a newspaper conveying the news, we hypothesise that maternal mental illness is a symptom of a wider group issue, be it from the present, or an intergenerational struggle.

At present, society situates the difficulty always in the individual. Is it the individual? Or is it a systemic failure? Motherhood is a time when women can feel mentally and physically unwell, anxious, stressed, overwhelmed and pressured. This is also when women need support to raise their child. We notice the continued negation of the importance of the mother, the lack of value attributed to mothering, the discounting and dismissal of the role of the mother. Instead, we see a system focused toward the individual, a system of blame, that continues to emphasise the individual mother as the container of the 'difficulty'. This discounts the importance of the system and thus reinforces this negative aspect. If the mother is seen as the representation of the system, she may be seen as an echo of the need for an echo chamber (system) to sustain life. Western society has become centred around the individual without attending to the echo system. The mother can be viewed as a representation of a dysfunctional system. However, we believe that the system ignores women and mothers and leaves them unsupported at our peril, as women hold an essential key to the future of humanity. At present, the women we see in our therapy rooms are often depleted, exhausted, ground down and struggling to bring up their children in the best way possible. If they ask for help from those agencies that are supposedly in place to support them – health services, social support agencies, governments – there is little or no provision for support. We see the 'mother' as depleted of energy and resources, and the maternal is similarly depleted. This has widespread implications, both societally and environmentally.

We argue that the quality of a human being's welfare hinges on the formation of protocol. Understanding how humans function and why they may think, feel and behave in particular ways requires knowledge of this foundational structure. Protocol is the essence of human being as it underpins and, therefore, frames how humans experience their environment. It is where psycho-development and psychopathology begin and, as said earlier, is formed relationally. It is from this developmental point that the infant begins to adapt, and this adaptation begins in utero, structurally with the turning on and off of our genetic coding through the process of epigenetics and maternal effects. It is also the point at which physis, our 'force of nature' towards growth and perfection, may be diminished, suppressed and cut off.

Often, we see mothers who, as infants, experienced their own mother's mental illness and who will also be at risk of passing this down to their child/children. Is this nature, i.e. passed genetically through DNA, or is it nurture, i.e. learnt behaviour – what we in TA might view as an attribution – for example, a message such as "maternal mental illness is what us women experience in this family"? We believe this is not an 'either/or', it is a 'both/and' and as such believe psychotherapeutic treatment can act as a transgenerational brake, allowing the mother to find a healthier place of being, for the sake of herself, her infant's future mental health and the health of the family surrounding her, who all bear the brunt of this distressing and debilitating condition.

If we can explore the role of protocol and the vital role of the mother, or maternal-other,[2] within this, we can offer possibility of how a newborn's protocol can be nourished to allow physis to materialise, to allow the newborn to fulfil its potential.

Being Born and Becoming

We are born 'from' the female (Cavarero, 1990; Jantzen, 2004) yet we are not necessarily cared for by our mothers. Being born is

> i) to begin to exist at a certain point in time by ii) coming into the world with and as a specific body, and in a given place, set of relationships, and situation in society, culture and history, while iii) doing so by way of being conceived and gestated in and then exiting from the womb.
>
> (Stone, 2019, p. 1)

Being born is also seen by Hannah Arendt, in her theory of natality (our condition of being born), as a time of our greatest potential, our newness and uniqueness "our capacity to initiate something new" (as cited in Totschnig, 2017, p. 328)

> with each one of us offering the possibility of the new – new actions, new thoughts, new abilities, newness. This newness is the human equivalent of a kind of "superpower" – humans have the capacity and possibility to influence and act as a catalyst of change.
>
> (Haynes, 2023, p. 71)

Aristotle coined the idea of tabula rasa (1994/429b), or 'clean slate' in translation from Latin, meaning that our mind is blank at birth and that all knowledge comes from experience or perception. This idea underpins a nature–nurture split in Western philosophy and psychotherapy, that privileges nurture (how we experience and perceive, which is mostly in relationship) over nature (what we are born with). This tradition of thought was followed by Freud and Berne, who emphasised what happens after birth as the key to understanding becoming, with little to no accounting for what is at the point of, or prior to being born (Aldridge & Stilman, 2023).

We hold a different view, that protocol is already present (to some extent) at birth, and therefore, do not believe that humans are born with a 'clean slate'. Instead, "our corporeal starting point is far from blank, and shapes the trajectory and quality of our lives in fundamental ways, and sometimes, defining whether we are born into privilege or oppression, even before we have taken our first breath" (Aldridge & Stilman, 2023). Does this mean we are doomed at birth? That the protocol offers a prede-termined outcome for what is to become of a person? That, despite best efforts, supportive conditions and good therapeutic process, we cannot really change what has been given at birth? It is an important question that needs reflection.

The point of being born marks the beginning of a physical, organismic separation from (m)other. It is the beginning of our becoming intra-personal units in an organismic and psychological sense, our journey to sustain life and potentially make something of it. Metaphorically, the cards that we are dealt with at that point will shape not only the outcome of the game, but the way that the cards are being played. Our origins affect what we become – they define the course by repetition (re-cycle) or generate a force that strives away from it (up-cycle) with varying degrees of success, as well as human and envi-ronmental cost. As body psychotherapist Keleman stated – "Life is a pro-cess of forming. There is a continual reshaping of our bodily-self, from the unformed infant to the formed adult. Either we live this forming unreflec-tively, or we volitionally participate in influencing our *inherited* responses" (Keleman & Adler, 2000, p. 50).

We propose that when it comes to becoming – the unfolding of a human being – both the capacity and the power to change are going to be shaped by what we are born with. Such is protocol: it contains the core issues and the potential for them to change and evolve.

Safety and Danger

We would suggest that protocol holds within it our earliest encoded experiences of safety and danger, perhaps as a primitive form of 'protection'. This might be primarily for species survival, a form of cellular, 'tissue' knowing perhaps, held on a sensate level prior to the development of the neocortex. If this is the case, then there is the possibility that this may impact human potential, physis and intuition. However, before we explore these impacts, we need to explore the way in which an infant's brain develops a little more fully.

Humans have a universal capacity to recognise danger and safety that spans intersections such as culture or ethnicity. It would be simplistic to believe that this capacity is inherent in our DNA; we believe it is more complex than this. Epigenetics suggests that the fetus is indeed primed for the environment they are likely to live in, and maternal effects are part of this survival strategy. We also know that danger and safety are perceived through our senses and are not cognitive due to the need to act instinctively and not waste time thinking.

Human brains grow from the earliest moments post conception and develop in a particular order in utero and then continue to evolve well into adulthood. By week ten (post-conception), the basic neural system is established (Konkel, 2018). This means that the functional brain develops in utero. However, the brain will continue to develop post-birth, going through its most intense 'explosion' of neural networks in the first year of human life, followed by an intense period of synaptic pruning by the end of the second year post-birth, precisely the same time span as the formation of protocol.

The central autonomic nervous system (sympathetic and parasympathetic divisions) is formed in utero and assists the fetus in its transitional development to enable the fetus for birth (Mulkey & Plessis, 2018). Functional MRI (fMRI) scans of fetuses in utero now show the exact moment at which a human fetus's brain develops its different senses. It is known that the three adaptive circuitry systems that humans develop occur in utero, in a particular order – immobilisation (freeze/shutdown) is the earliest to develop (at around nine weeks post conception), followed by mobilisation (fetal locomotor activity) which is thought to develop around 16–20 weeks gestation, with the final, socialisation system developing just before birth allowing an infant to vocalise or grimace at birth; although Porges states that the vagal system is only partially functioning at birth (Porges, 2011). Danger activates the sympathetic nervous system and triggers an acute stress response – fight, flight or freeze. The brain develops in this way, almost certainly due to the need for human survival, vital for the survival of the species and therefore this cellular development will be held within our DNA.

Within the first year, post-birth, there is a literal explosion of synapses occurring within the infant's brain. Synaptic pruning is also vital and is relevant to protocol. Within these first two years, an infant's brain distinguishes between the 'important' connections and those less important (those synapses that are not used), to prune away the 'unimportant', for cognitive efficiency. The brain removes all of the inefficient, unused pathways, so that the connectome – the billions of labyrinthine neural connections across the brain that signal to each other, which some believe form our behaviour, personality, cognition and memory (Konkel, 2018) – works as efficiently as possible. Thus, this is the time when an infant is most vulnerable to environmental and/ or maternal stress factors. Neglect or lack of interaction between a maternal-other and her infant in these crucial first two years of development may mean the loss of vital neural pathways. Responsive relationships are fundamental for the development of human brain circuitry. The infant may reach out, coo or form facial expressions, and needs a response to these to shape and develop their brain. Therefore, a lack of interaction or neglect may mean the pruning away of those neurons regarding connection, relationship, speech and language formation, and some of the most fundamental building blocks of development, such as basic hand-to-eye coordination, which may impact their learning, their behaviour and also health going forward.

> Because responsive relationships are both expected and essential, their absence is a serious threat to a child's development and well-being. Sensing threat activates biological stress response systems and excessive activation of those systems can have a toxic effect on developing brain circuitry. When the lack of responsiveness persists, the adverse effects of toxic stress can compound the lost opportunities for development associated with limited or ineffective interaction. This multifaceted impact of neglect on the developing brain underscores why it is so harmful in the earliest years of life and why effective early interventions are likely to pay significant dividends in better, long-term outcomes in educational achievement, lifelong health, and successful parenting of the next generation.
>
> (Centre on the Developing Child, 2013)

The regulatory process also begins in utero; the mother regulates the fetus through biological and affective processes, "a continuum... between the infant's pre-natal and post-natal life: the caregiver continues to regulate the infant's affective life" (Taipale, 2016, p. 4). DiPietro, Costigan and Voegtline conceptualise this as an involvement between fetus and pregnant woman that is reciprocal and "spiralling" (2015, p. 7). A fetus/infant responds to the 'mother' with either a soothed or a heightened somatic experience. Taipale states this is not true "co-regulation", and instead highlights a "pre-dyadic" regulatory process first (2016). This pre-dyadic regulatory process begins a process of 'remembering' that forms the foundation of "patterns of affect regulation that integrate a sense of self across state transitions, hereby allowing for a continuity of inner experience" (Schore, 1994, p. 33). Pre-dyadic regulation is when there is no distinguishment in the infant between how the infant's self feels and how the 'other' feels (Taipale, 2016, p. 4).

> In favourable circumstances, the newborn infant gradually attaches to the caregiver: she begins to favour, seek into, and desire for, this peculiar, increasingly differentiated experiential presence that, in her experience is, with increasing precision, associated with affective balance and well-being. However, even if the caregiver's affective presence is increasingly differentiated from the presence of other affective sources – the former might not yet be clearly differentiated from the infant herself ... During times of need, the caregiver plays the function of a regulative shield and she might not be experienced as being anything more than that.
>
> (Taipale, 2016, p. 5)

With time and repetition this becomes a 'knowing' of somatic, affective and cognitive states of safety and danger. Taipale draws attention to infants "catching the mood" of those around them – "babies tend to feel distressed when people around them are distressed, and they tend to feel calmer when people around them are calm" (2016, p. 4). Trauma is what we call the interruptions to this process of experience that becomes knowledge. These interruptions shape future decoding of experiences, in that the decoding of safety and danger is also interrupted and, therefore, furthers the interrupted states of safety and danger. It's a self-fulfilling recursive process. Trauma seems to be able to penetrate protocol, probably because protocol operates at the subsymbolic level – the sensory, affective, somatic and motor modes of mental processing (Cornell, 2008a). Caizzi (2012) believes protocol can be changed due to extreme negative relational experiences such as torture or extreme trauma, wherein the violation occurs to the individual's body at such a level that it penetrates through the body's safety and defence system. We do not have enough space here to open up this area of trauma and how it would penetrate protocol.

Taipale's research has enhanced knowledge of the first period, post-birth, of an infant's life, where "the pressing need organizes the infant's whole experiential reality, and the caregiver is initially nothing more than what [they are] in the light of the infant's current needs and wants". This helps with understanding how in the pre-dyadic regulation: "the infant does not yet distinguish between **how [they themselves] feel** and **how the other feels**" (2016, p. 4, emphasis in the original text). This differentiating self from other is important and protocol, the time during which there is the capacity for this to occur, is vital – because this is the foundation stone of self-regulation. What Taipale states helps transactional analysts to consider the time span of the formation of ego states and when the self can differentiate between that of the other. In Chapter 6, this is expanded a little.

The knowledge of brain formation in utero and within the first two years post-birth has updated the way in which science now understands the capacity of a fetus and infant within its first days and weeks of life, and has required an update to, for example, the care and attention that infants need. What this shows transactional analysis theory is that protocol warrants more appraisal and research, and we will endeavour to explain why as we explore protocol in more depth. However, prior to this we need to delve a little into Berne's thinking about protocol.

Transactional Analytic Theory of Protocol: a Critique

The most influential writers on protocol are firstly Berne, then Cornell and Landaiche, who updated Berne's theory in their 2006 article "Impasse and Intimacy: Applying Berne's Concept of Script Protocol", and finally Cornell himself who stated protocol may be now seen more as "implicit, procedural memory" (2019, p. 6).

Berne first wrote about protocol in 1961 and used the term to describe "the earliest version of script incorporating the earliest memories and decisions *with our earliest relational figures*" (Tilney, 1998, p. 95, our emphasis). For Berne, protocol represented the first household drama and was formed in the earliest part of our lives, from birth to around 2 or 3 years of age, when he believed protocol was superseded by script proper. He described protocol as "played out to an unsatisfactory conclusion in the earliest years of life … Its precipitates re-appear as the 'script proper', which is a preconscious derivative of the protocol" (1961, p. 117). Berne's thinking around protocol seemed to be born out of his exploration of 'intuition' and, in particular, from one paper "Intuition IV: Primal Images and Primal Judgements" (1955/1977a). Berne believed that, initially, an infant was only able to store feelings as an anonymous "image", due to the infant's lack of language, and that the infant would then form a "judgement" about that image. "In essence, a primal image is an impression made on the child's body by a significant other's 'mode of relating'" (Berne, 1955, p. 68). Cornell and Landaiche (2006) understood this as

> a cluster of sensations, organized outside awareness by the child, that reflects his or her experience of another before the child has access to words or symbols. Berne considered the child's organising role to be an act of primal judgment, similar to the judgments we make about our worlds throughout life and, in particular, about others we see as allies or enemies.
>
> (2006, p. 202)

Cornell and Landaiche saw behaviours based on protocol as "deeply compelling, implicit (wordless) memory of primary relational patterns lived through the immediacy of bodily experience" (2006, p. 203). They did not see these as necessarily pathological and this is an important point which we will come back to.

Briefly, returning to Berne, he called the primal image the "pre-symbolic, non-verbal representation of interpersonal transactions" (1977a, p. 67) upon which the infant based his "primal judgement". As Cornell and Landaiche point out, Berne saw these (the primal images and primal judgements) as simultaneous processes. Berne also described a "tissue level" (1975/1972, p. 111) of experience which Cornell differentiated from script protocol, calling it "third-degree script" (2008a, p. 162). Mellacqua believes that this would be viewed now as "implicit memory or subsymbolic organization" (2021, p. 78). We will explore implicit memory in a moment.

Furthermore, Cornell and Landaiche wrote of protocols "as ongoing, unconscious templates for making judgements about the significant figures and encounters in our lives" (2005, p. 19). Whilst we agree with Cornell and Landaiche, that protocol is a cluster of sensations and perhaps a somatic memory – a blurring of sensations (smelt, touched, heard, felt, seen, etc.) that is held within the body as part of our threat response, which may or may not be helpful – we question the usefulness of the words 'image' and 'judgement'. We prefer to think of it as an encoded response, rather than either an image or judgement.

Returning to implicit memory for a moment and what it actually comprises, implicit memory can be called "non-declarative memory, motor memory or procedural memory, and it cannot be described in words. For this memory to form, overt conscious appreciation of memory is not necessary" (Dharani, 2015, p. 53). Implicit memory guides our interpersonal relationships; it is this that pulls us towards or pushes us away from particular 'others' and although it is 'memory' it is not cognitive memory and is stored in areas of the brain in which memories cannot be retrieved due to the developmental stage in which the memory is formed.

In their article "Nonconscious Processes and Self-Development: Key Concepts from Berne and Bollas" (2008), Cornell and Landaiche highlight Mancia's (2004/2007) idea of implicit memory as the store of nonconscious materials such as priming (visual/auditory recognition of an object), procedural memory (our numerous unconscious motor and cognitive abilities used nonconsciously – riding a bicycle, playing sports, making a cup of tea), and emotional affective memory (our earliest affective memories of our environment, in particular our mother). Cornell and Landaiche highlight the importance of the interpersonal element of the nonconscious, not just the cognitive/emotional processes, which fits with our emphasis on the relational aspect of protocol.

Pierini, in her 2008 article "Has the Unconscious Moved House?" also drew our attention to implicit knowledge, which she called "nonverbal and analogue" (p. 112), adding Stern's (2005) formulation of implicit knowledge: "not in the realm of awareness but it is not repressed; it has just never been conscious" (p. 28). For Pierini, the term "nonconscious" modernises the psychoanalytic term 'unconscious' and is more appropriate in transactional analytic theory because it recognises the existence of various processing systems (neuronal, emotional and subsymbolic) that are at work outside of awareness: "The term 'nonconscious' takes into account the outcome of implicit knowledge and its related implicit memory, which also preserves pleasant experiences that no one would want to remove" (p. 111). The nonconscious would include experiences from preverbal, presymbolic developmental stages. Pierini goes on to quote Allen (2003), who stated that implicit memories "are not available to conscious autobiographical memory, although they control the capacity to invest in and to share with others, are of major importance in staying alive, procreating, and protecting and nurturing the young" (p. 131). Both Allen and Pierini drew our attention to the importance of these first attachment relationships which are part of protocol, as they are the foundation stones of our belief systems, about self, others and the world around us and are vital to our survival. We agree with Pierini and her concept of the nonconscious, which is why this is used in preference to the unconscious within this chapter.

Erskine hinted at protocol in his definition of life scripts: "Life scripts are a complex set of unconscious relational patterns based on physiological survival reactions, implicit experiential conclusions, explicit decisions and/or self-regulating introjections" (Erskine, 2010a, p. 1). Within his description of effective change in the life script he stated: "being aware of the client's bodily reactions and uncovering the unconscious emotional story embedded within his or her body" (Erskine, 2010b). His reference to the implicit and the unconscious is important, as is his reference to these being 'embedded' within the body.

Mellacqua, in his book *Transactional Analysis of Schizophrenia: The Naked Self* (2021), which focuses on the treatment of psychotic disorders using his innovative ideas steeped in TA theory, highlights protocol as the earliest relational patterns and talks of script, as Berne did, as an updated version of the crude, first version of script, with its origins in "the earliest infant period" (p. 20). But what is the earliest infant period? Is it post-birth, or is it in utero or both? Mellacqua sees protocol as the "always active sensed, polysensory, interbodily, nonconscious and nonverbal dimension of human experience of being and being in relation to someone" (p. 21), where there is not a formed differentiation between self and other, yet. We agree with this perception of the lack of the formed differentiation between self and other, as stated earlier, due to the research of Joona Taipale. In his book, Mellacqua also appears to point to protocol beginning to form in utero:

> Everything that happens before the individual assumes a more conscious existential I–You position is related to the ineffable and early

neonatal (even intrauterine) and infant period of life, during which nonverbal, preverbal and unconscious relationship experiences are formed between the individual and primary caregiving figures.

(2021, p. 20)

Why did Berne use the term protocol? If we look at a dictionary definition of this word, its meaning focuses around rules and acceptable behaviour or formal agreements between governments (i.e. the Kyoto protocol). In computer science, it is used as a set of rules defining the structure and manner of exchange of information between devices in computer networks. If we consider the brain as a neural network, and family or society as a set of neural networks, then we could hypothesise that protocol (as a set of encoded rules) helps us decipher what is safe and what is dangerous, including recognising in others safety and danger threat responses. Whilst in the earliest TA theory, the term 'protocol' did not gain particular attention, Berne astutely realised that an infant was storing its earliest experiences and 'memories' at a cellular (tissue) level rather than a cognitive level during those youngest years of life. These then influence the infant's life position and script and continue to influence the infant (nonconsciously or preconsciously) for the entirety of its life.

Transgenerational Protocol

We suggest that individuals hold memory of their conception, gestation and birth at a cellular level and want to share our thinking in how we see this relating to transactional analysis theory.

As stated above, the environment in utero and externally for the pregnant mother is fundamental in the shaping of protocol. Protocol forms inter-relationally and a fetus 'marinades' within the environment, which flows through and around the placenta and the fetus in utero, via the mother. This amniotic fluid, which we could think of as the fetus's first environment, is filled with all the gases and hormones needed to support growth. However, some hormones, such as those caused by stress and toxins, are also part of the amniotic fluid and would also impact the fetus through epigenetic processes, modifying gene presentation (see Carey, 2012 for a thorough review of epigenetics). However, in our view protocol begins forming much earlier than birth. In fact, we would suggest that it could already exist on a cellular basis within transgenerational evolutionary scripting in what we call "transgenerational protocol".

We argue that to communicate survival needs, aspects of protocol are passed down through the generations. TA authors have written about transgenerational trauma (Hargaden, 2016; Gayol, 2004; Novak, 2013, 2022; Stuthridge & Rowland, 2019). However, we do not believe the transgenerational is only about trauma being passed down generationally. We believe that we all carry an ancestral cellular 'knowing'. This idea was also highlighted by McQuillin and Welford (2013) and alluded to by Apprey who described the process of "transgenerational haunting" as "sedimentations of history" (p. 344). As such, we would like to open up dialogue around how the maternal can inform us of this transgenerational evolutionary passing on of survival knowledge: be it hauntings, needs, mandates, strategies or aspirations.

This idea goes beyond the transferential domain and is not science fiction, but firmly rooted in genetics. It is common knowledge that the paternal chromosome 'Y' is passed through the male lineage and determines the gender of the fetus. This means that paternal lineage is maintained as long as the fetus is male. However, a more interesting phenomenon that could illustrate a strong link between transgenerational 'knowing' and the maternal, is the mitochondrial DNA. The mitochondrial DNA is passed exclusively through the maternal lineage irrespective of the fetus gender. This distinct DNA structure is unique to the maternal lineage and is not mixed with the paternal DNA. The mitochondrial DNA acts as the cell's power source and is responsible for converting chemical energy from food into a form that a cell can use. The sperm is created with a small amount of mitochondrial DNA that is only enough for the sperm to travel onto the egg. The egg, however, is created with an abundance of mitochondrial DNA that persists through the creation of the egg, insemination and development into a fetus.

Berne informed us of the need to consider "the influence of the grandparents" (Berne, 1975/1972, p. 288). Considering the above, however, we would argue to account for much more than just the grandparent generation. It is the environment our ancestors grew up in that may still be impacting us in the present moment, and humans may find it impossible to articulate or to 'know' what that environment was. As transgenerational protocol may be nonconscious, and nonverbal, carried at a sensate and cellular level only (Haynes, 2023), it is not part of cognition and is not part of the neocortex. It would, therefore, be impossible to think oneself out of being in it. We have been spurred into writing about and opening up dialogue around protocol more fully because we believe transgenerational protocol and the environment in which it was formed (at conception, gestation and birth) is key not only in understanding the lifelong adverse impact it has on ourselves and our clients, but is also a way to tap into the potential that they are born with.

Berne used the term physis to give a name to the way in which humans are genetically programmed to survive and thrive. Taking our thoughts further, are protocol and potential the difference between survival and thriving? We do not necessarily have an answer to this question, yet there may be a paradox in not having a 'tabula rasa' and being born with potential. If humans are born with potential, what is needed for that potential to materialise? Some may attribute this 'needed' element to the controversial nurture versus nature debate (Galton, 1875). Is it more important to nurture, to focus on parenting in a way that allows the infant to thrive with good early childhood experiences and to provide an environment conducive to positive experiences both socially and culturally when growing and developing? Or is it about nature, our genetics, not only the genes we are born with, but also those hereditary genes, elements that some may believe are natural regardless of influences from the environment during gestation, birth and our development? This book is situated in the nurture position, advocating for mothers to gain the support they require to do the best job they can in raising the next generation. We wonder whether it is a highly complex and individual combination of the two, nature and nurture.

Is protocol only about surviving, while potential is about thriving? How might the struggle to survive get in the way of thriving? How may the past experience of survival of our ancestors passed on a cellular level, encoding how they learnt to move, act, speak, behave in a way that was imperative for their survival 'back then', serve or interfere with fulfilling potential in the present? In his attempt to understand sociological changes of the post-modern world, Wagner coined the idea of the dialectic of progress (1993) as a way of accounting for the inevitable destructiveness that human development encompasses; perhaps this illustrates best the paradoxical tension that lies within protocol – how can the creative endeavour of human survival transform to thriving? And what might not survive to sustain this thriving?

Protocol, Intuition and Creativity

Let's turn to protocol, intuition and creativity and explore whether there is an interaction between these three and how this interaction may occur, if it does. Perhaps it is easiest to begin by exploring intuition. Berne defined intuition as "knowledge based on experience and acquired through sensory contact with the subject, without the 'intuiter' being able to formulate to himself or others exactly how he came to his conclusions" (1949/1977b, p. 4). Many different schools of psychology have offered up as many definitions of intuition. On closer inspection it would appear a controversial area in psychology due to the need to pin down a concept with empirical research evidence. As such, intuition has proven to be a slippery concept. For the purpose of this chapter, we use a humanistic and transactional analytic lens and understand intuition as a nonconscious mode of knowing (a judgement – both cognitive and affective) which occurs rapidly without conscious knowledge of how that judgement was made. This is somewhat akin to Bollas's "unthought known" (1987). Returning to our view of protocol, we believe some of this intuition or unthought known is located within script protocol.

In mathematics, as in music, the capacity and freedom for intuition is developed through repetition and practice. The repetition increases the flow and accuracy of identifying and applying patterns in calculation, expression and, ultimately, improvisation. Each time we improvise, we learn and that becomes part of the pattern as it expands in permutations. The same applies to human behaviour. Humans are creatures of pattern, and with time these patterns, shaped and informed by protocol, become deeply ingrained in implicit memory, or "unconscious competence" (Broadwell, 1969), so that the person can apply them without thought. These form the basis of how to respond to situations by following a pattern, and when an unknown situation emerges where an existing pattern does not apply, an approximation needs to be quickly improvised. This is where the concept of intuition becomes useful. One's body communicates a sense of how to go about the foreign situation that is not fully formulated. It is a feeling of how to go about this, possibly much closer to a "primal judgement" than Berne intended. Once formulated and tested, it moves from intuition into capacity.

Moving on to creativity, Haynes (2022) defined creativity as a "tripartite definition of novelty and effectiveness (Cropley, 2011) as well as originality (Andreason, 2011)" (p. 136) and wrote about other transactional analysts who have explored the connection between intuition and creativity such as Chiesa (2012a, 2012b, 2014) and Cornell (2010, 2011). Haynes has already drawn attention to the use of creative methods in practice in psychotherapy, working with the maternal and the way in which she believes this can help psychotherapists to step into the unknown with clients and in particular unlock silence, or silent aspects of the therapy. Creativity and what it offers perinatal psychotherapy will be explored in Chapter 8.

Within TA, there is a widely positive regard to the ideas of intuition and creativity. Intuition is seen as some sort of expression of our natural tendency for contact and growth, of our humanity, and in TA we are often encouraged to trust our intuition or foster a capacity for paying attention to intuition when it is shut down or killed off. Creativity is seen also as a huge asset to humans due to the impact and richness it can have on the arts, innovation and science (MacKinnon, 1962; Ritter et al., 2020).

Yet, if intuition and creativity are also informed by protocol – as patterns passed on through the generation to aid survival, might it also mean that our ways of decoding safety and danger can be out of context for the environment in which we are present? And if so, how can intuition and creativity be regarded as so positive? Could it be that our intuition could ultimately lead to more pain and suffering or even get in the way of thriving? How can we know that our intuition is wise knowledge? Pondering on the impact of trauma within the earliest moments of life – developmental trauma – combined with continued early traumatic formative experiences, and the influence this may have on intuition and creativity throughout life, what if intuition is thwarted or warped in some way that draws the person towards danger rather than turning them away from it?

Thinking also about the idea within epigenetics that a person's experiences (both from childhood or within adulthood) might alter their biology and behaviour, as well as the way their genes are expressed, and that this may be inherited through three generations, then Berne's words: "The most intricate part of script analysis in clinical practice is tracing back the influences of the grandparents" (p. 288) becomes even more vital. How many trainee TA psychotherapists are taught the need to take such a detailed assessment of their client? Perhaps this is what Apprey means when he talks about "early and deep" (2019, p. 342), which we take to mean the impact on the infant of the earliest developmental processes and the lasting and profound impact they have on the infant's entire life. Perhaps in some contexts, our intuition and creativity could be almost delusional. It might be a combination of both. If we take the extreme example of the holocaust – trusting the humanity of others led a few to survive by trusting in the goodwill of strangers. For many others, it cost them their lives. Conversely, those who did not trust others may have resulted in them attempting to escape or retaliate, with equally varying degrees of mortality. What we find helpful to consider by this illustration is that our potential can be counterintuitive to our survival protocol.

Conclusion

This chapter is complex and filled with a dense level of thought and theory. However, the concept of script protocol is so important, not only within TA theory but also within the concept of the maternal, that we have felt the need to delve deeply into it. It is important to start from Berne, followed by a brief review of the most important and significant writing that updated what was quite a scant offering from Berne on this area. However, as with many of his theories, it is actually quite incredible how much foresight Berne afforded us in his writing on protocol, a concept that does not seem to exist in the same manner within other modalities of psychotherapy. We are grateful to Berne for his foresight.

Our aim in writing this chapter together was to offer insight into the relevance of protocol within maternal mental health, as a way of encouraging more research and theory on this influential area, as well as to encourage more psychotherapists to work in this area. We also believe that our thoughts on protocol may have relevance to the three other fields of transactional analysis, as pregnancy, birth and parenting are a significant part of every human's life, even if they choose not to tread onto the parenting pathway. Every human was in utero, and we may be impacted by those around us who are going through what can be such a difficult struggle, even if it is only within the work or friendship space. If pregnancy, birth and parenting are considered as a metaphor of systemic components of any liminal process, these concepts can easily be applied to organisations, education and change in its entire human aspect.

We have shown how protocol is formed in utero at the same moment that very particular parts of brain development relating to safety and danger are formed, and the negative and positive connotations this may have for an infant. We have also highlighted how protocol could impact three elements of life both positively and negatively – physis, potential and intuition – and how these may offer a key to understanding the difference between surviving and thriving. The potential a newborn offers is huge, yet there is a lack of appreciation and support for the maternal in conceiving, carrying, delivering and bringing up the infant in a way that allows the release of this potential. We hope we are in a time where this may begin to shift in terms of social and economic affordance, knowledge and understanding to a more collaborative and complementary set of functions that engender the release of the potential of as many infants as possible and minimise the adverse and limiting impact of the transgenerational passing on of protocol without diminishing its potential and value. For the sake of the next generations of parents and infants, our Mother Earth and the sake of humanity itself.

Notes

1 Whenever the term 'we' is used within this chapter it means both of us, Emma and Ronen.
2 Throughout this chapter, we have chosen to use the term maternal-other in order to encompass 'care-giver', 'maternal', 'mother'. We do not wish to pathologise all 'mothers'.

6

THE FUNDAMENTAL ROLE OF 'MOTHER' IN AN INFANT'S LIFE

Attachment and Affect Regulation

The 'other' is the foundation of human life. Even prior to conception, others form us through their egg and sperm. Regardless of whether these 'others' remain a part of our lives, humans, from conception, are in relationship with others. Everything humans learn about themselves in space and time is due to the other. This other might mean anything, and may be an object, an animal, an environment or a plant, for example, as these are all important in an infant's journey towards differentiating self from other. The most critical others are of course humans, who fulfil our relational needs. Berne recognised these needs and called them "hungers" – for recognition, stimulus, contact, sex, time structure and incident hunger (Berne, 1970). Recognition, stimulus and structure hunger (Berne, 1961) are pivotal in an infant's life and are dependent on 'mother', so let's delve more deeply into this first fundamental relationship and explore the role of 'mother' and why so much of life and health hinges on it.

Attachment and affect regulation are the foundation stones of human relationships, very much interrelated, and fundamentally interlinked with good enough mothering, a concept first written about in 1971 by Donald Winnicott. Having a secure attachment style and the ability to self-regulate are essential to a person's capacity to thrive rather than simply survive, and these two elements are key components in the difference between mental health and a person's predisposition to mental ill health. Affect regulation is a learned skill shown, through neuroscientific research, to begin almost certainly before birth. It then continues to develop through childhood well into adulthood. This skill is most often learnt from the mother due to the length of time she spends with her infant and their intense connection.

How we attached to our parents in childhood and how they helped us to self-soothe plays a vital part in how we are with our children. When the attachment process is upset and insecure, the parent may struggle with attachment and find it challenging to offer a calm and nurturing environment to their infant. Being nurtured and soothed may be a void in their knowledge. One helpful element of relational psychotherapy is how it can help enhance and

DOI: 10.4324/9781003365822-6

change a parent's capacity to self-regulate, helping them to tolerate adversity and painful emotions. As Alan Schore states:

> Although early relationships shape the developing brain, the human brain remains plastic and capable of learning throughout the entire lifespan, and with the right therapeutic help we can move beyond dissociation as our primary defence mechanism and begin to regulate our emotions more appropriately.
>
> (Schore, 2019, pp. 241–242)

Schore offers a great deal of hope for those embarking on relational psychotherapy, something he advocates in his 2019 publication – *Right Brain Psychotherapy*.

Self-regulation helps us with our social connections, is part of emotional intelligence, and helps us to build the capacity for tolerance. When a person can self-regulate, they have the ability to deal with adversity and disappointment and control any negative impulses as a reaction to uncomfortable feelings. However, according to research by Burman, Green and Shanker in 2015, one of the most common features that seems to be missing in many psychotherapy clients is the ability to self-regulate. I certainly see many clients who find regulating their emotions extremely difficult. It would appear that a lack of affect regulation is often missed when considering the possible underlying causes of mental illness.

I have also noticed how many of the parents I see confuse good enough with perfect parenting. Many of my clients show extreme anxiety, particularly around their own parenting ability due to their limited ability to self-regulate. This may then hinder or limit them in regulating their infant, leading to a transgenerational lack or absence of emotional regulation and a possible heritable transmission of negative emotions such as anxiety and fear. Not only this, a parent with an insecure attachment may struggle to create the required environment in which their infant can become securely attached. I am not for a moment suggesting that all parents with insecure attachment struggle to be 'good enough' parents or, indeed, cannot securely attach to their children. I am saying that this may prove more challenging, and hence those who are challenged may come into psychotherapy seeking help.

In Chapter 5, I highlighted the importance of the earliest experiences between mother and infant due to the explosion in infant brain development during pregnancy and within the first three years of life. This chapter will expand on this knowledge to show the essential role of the 'other' – the mother/caregiver – highlighting mirroring and attunement and the role these play in infant interpersonal understanding, differentiation and social recognition. These three – interpersonal understanding, differentiation and social recognition – help an infant with the vital task of forming a sense of self. Disruptions in the attachment system and in affect regulation from neglect and/or childhood trauma and abuse lead to a lack of mirroring and attune-ment, which thwart a child's ability to develop interpersonal abilities and to understand others' and their own mental states (Ball Cooper et al., 2021) and therefore disrupt them gaining a coherent sense of self.

For the purpose of clarity, bonding and attachment are often used as if they were synonymous, yet there are distinct differences between them. Kraemer (1992) gives four essential elements in attachment theory:

1   An infant is born with inbuilt behaviours towards the 'mother' thus attachment is instinctive, not learned, nor reinforced.
2   Attachment maintains the child's perception of safety and security, through protection by the caregiver (Bowlby, 1982).
3   Attachment gives internal representations of 'mother' and their environ-ment which the infant uses to 'predict' the behaviour of others and to regulate their behaviour.
4   The secure base – offered by 'mother' allows the infant to explore, subject to homeostasis (Ettenberger et al., 2021).

Attachment is not bonding. The term bonding comes from the research of Klaus and Kennell in the 1970s (Klaus & Kennell, 1970; Kennell & Klaus, 1984) and is controversial.

> Attachment theory describes essentially how the child builds up a relationship with its primary caregiver and bonding theory describes the feelings, thoughts, and behaviors of the parent towards the baby. Thus, they focus on different sides of the early parent–infant relationship.
>
> (Ettenberger et al., 2021, S. 3.3)

Benoit (2004) states that research shows no connection between bonding and any positive or negative child outcomes and that attachment does show this connection and also predicts the child's social and emotional outcomes pow-erfully. However, new longitudinal research (Le Bas et al., 2020) shows posi-tive developmental benefits of a good mother-to-baby bond between the ages of 0 and 24 months.

Self-regulation is the capacity and ability to manage our thoughts, emo-tions, behaviour and how we react to different experiences and events. In this chapter I will mainly talk about self-regulation as there is no room to elabo-rate the discussion into the area of mentalization (Fonagy et al., 1991), a capacity beyond self-regulation, which is the ability to understand not only our own thoughts, beliefs, wishes and feelings (i.e. mental states), and how they are linked to our behaviour, but also those of others. It is theorised by Ball Cooper et al. that this lack of attachment security and mentalizing abil-ity may be the basis for all psychopathology (2021). I also see much from the theories of mentalization which might be interlinked and integrated with Pio Scilligo's concept of the Integrated Self (2009). However, this is out of the scope of this book and must wait for another day.

Good Enough Mothering

When parents struggle, some of their difficulties may come from the burden of striving for perfection in their parenting ability. This can be driven by parenting myths, peer and family pressure, and social media, among other things, that may push them to strive for perfection in themselves and their infant. However, they might not realise that being the 'perfect' parent is detrimental to an infant's mental well-being and is impossible to maintain because no parent can remain empathic, available and responsive at all times. Equally, some parents simply have no concept of good parenting or grew up with abusive, harmful parents and may unknowingly continue this cycle of abuse, neglect and/or harm transgenerationally.

Donald Winnicott, the famous paediatrician, wrote about what he termed as 'good enough mothering' in his book *Playing and Reality*: "The good-enough mother is one who makes active adaptation to the infant's needs, an active adaptation that gradually lessens, according to the infant's growing ability to account for failure of adaptation and to tolerate the results of frustration" (Winnicott, 1971, p. 7).

It is the mother or primary caregiver who "to a large extent maintains affect regulation on behalf of the infant: the caregiver is initially not just in the service of the infant's affect regulation, but rather in charge of it" (Taipale, 2016). This is because when an infant has needs – food, a nappy change, calming – the infant is engulfed by that need, and does not care about how the need is fulfilled nor the mood of the person fulfilling it. In fact, infants have the ability to show that the need is one of life and death through the intensity of their cry: "The pressing need organizes the infant's whole experiential reality, and the caregiver is initially nothing more than what she is in light of the infant's current needs and wants" (Taipale, 2016).

Although good enough mothering has been known about for 50+ years, I believe it is apparent that this concept is not readily understood. Also, in his writing, Winnicott used the term mother yet acknowledged that this was not only the biological mother. This is important. I have placed the word mother in quotes in the title of this chapter because the meaning of this word means more than biological mother and would include a foster, step and adoptive parent, as well as the primary caregiver.

The Intertwining of Attachment and Affect Regulation

Affects – our emotions – are fundamentally important. When an infant is born, there is an intensity in the bond between the caregiver, usually the mother, and the infant. There is also a myriad of emotions within that intense bond – love all the way through to rage, and even terror when there is fear of loss of attachment. As stated previously, affect regulation and attachment begin before birth, and what we are taught about these in childhood tends to remain with us through life, which may be why change in both can seem so difficult, if not impossible. Alan Schore (2019), an expert in human development, discovered that attachment promotes self-regulation and this in turn allows for new and more complex and resilient relational interactions between the person and their social environment. From infancy and throughout the whole of our lives, spontaneous, rapidly acting emotional processes that are generated in our right brain hemisphere are fundamental in enabling the person to regulate and thereby manage with the stresses and challenges they encounter throughout their life.

For theorists from an attachment perspective, secure attachment would equal good affect regulation, underlining the intertwining of the two concepts. Within psychoanalysis, affect regulation is also important, and the belief is that good affect regulation can lead to self-regulation (Fonagy et al., 2004), a higher self-understanding ability through appraisal, informational processing and attention towards affects.

Self-regulation means being capable of choosing to change our emotional state or the ability to mentalize – reflecting upon the emotional state – as a new way of relating to and gaining control over our emotions. In 1994 Schore argued that "the core of the self lies in patterns of affect regulation that integrate a sense of self across state transitions, thereby allowing for a continuity of inner experience" (p. 33). Within TA, we may theorise that a person who can regulate themselves in the manner Schore describes above might be deemed to be in their integrating Adult ego state (Tudor, 2003), as the integrating Adult is described as having the ability to self-regulate while experiencing heightened affects.

However, at this point, it is also important to acknowledge that self-regulation is not easy to achieve, nor can it be maintained permanently. It can be all too easy to mistake and misunderstand emotions in ourselves and in others.

The Importance of 'Mother' in Regulatory Processes

A mother needs to be preoccupied with her infant from birth for those very first months of life. This is totally natural, as an infant requires devotional care from a person who is absolutely adapted symbiotically to their needs. At this point in life, an infant has absolutely no capacity for self-regulation and relies entirely on the caregiver to regulate them. In Figure 6.1, I have shown in diagrammatic form what I consider to be the basic infant developmental stages, which I have combined with the primary role of the caregiver. I have chosen to use a triangle to represent these three fundamental stages of

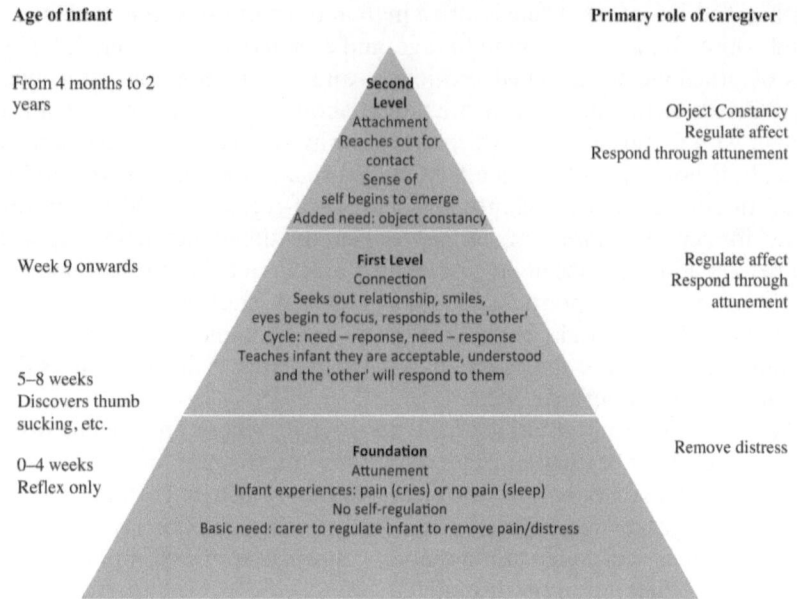

Figure 6.1 The Primary Role of the Caregiver

development because I wish to give a sense of the stages being built, one upon the other, almost like a set of children's building blocks.

The first stage of an infant's post-birth life is what I call the Foundation because I see this as the foundational stage of infant development, and it is onto this stage that attachment and affect regulation can begin to form and develop. During this foundation period, an infant is either asleep (satiated, with no pressing need) or awake and often crying due to discomfort (from hunger perhaps or a dirty nappy) and needing someone to respond to them by taking away their discomfort. During these first few weeks in an infant's life, there are very few moments when an infant is awake and in a state of 'alert inactivity' (Wolf, 1966; Stern, 1977, 1985). This is almost certainly due to the immense amount of growth the infant goes through, both bodily and within its brain and organs, requiring the infant to sleep most of the time when not feeding. During this foundational stage, the infant's basic need is for the carer to regulate the infant by removing any pain and distress. The person who is doing the caregiving may not be quite so vital or important in these four weeks. What is more pressing is that the infant is responded to and attended to and can return to sleep feeling satiated and comfortable.

In Figure 6.1, the stage above Foundation is what I call the First Level. This is when an infant begins to show signs of connection with the caregiver. Around about 5–8 weeks, some infants will discover their thumb (some may have discovered this already) and, therefore, have some rudimentary form of self-regulation. Some parents will use a dummy as another form of regulation at this early stage. But other than these rudimentary forms, the infant still utterly relies on the primary caregiver for regulation.

At around 8–9 weeks post-birth, the infant begins to seek connection through smiling and responding to the caregiver, and their eyes begin to focus on people or things close to them. They begin to gain a better sense of people and things around them, because they are more able to see, particularly at the distance of an adult arm, which is around 25 cm. The baby can now track objects with their eyes and can recognise the caregiver's face. They will also begin to reach for things and can see colour (Nationwide Children's Hospital, 2023). This is the beginning of what I call the need–response cycle. Although this cycle was present in the Foundation level, it is during this First Level, the beginning of connection, that the primary caregiver becomes much more important. The infant has a need and will cry out for the 'other' to respond to that need. If the primary caregiver can regulate the infant and respond to their needs through attunement, this begins the process of teaching the infant that they are acceptable, that the 'other' (the primary caregiver) understands their need and that they will be responded to. This is the basic foundation for attachment.

The final level at this basic stage of infant development is what I call the Second Level in Figure 6.1 and is the beginning of proper attachment. It is a time when an infant begins to require object constancy. What I mean by object constancy is that the primary caregiver remains the constant safe and secure presence within the infant's life, which is itself a regulatory process as the infant can seek refuge with this secure presence (Bretherton, 1992). An infant with different caregivers coming and going may not gain any semblance of safety and security, as there may be little constancy and continuity in its young life. Infants with little in the way of object constancy can show signs of extreme distress when the primary caregiver leaves, or may become quiet, distant and disconnected. If the infant is continually not attended to through regulation in these instances, and is left unregulated in most times of distress, this can have a severe negative impact: "If she is left to deal with demanding affective situations by herself, the outcome tends to be dramatic – e.g. in an overtly stressful environment, a baby might withdraw psychologically and fall into apathy" (Taipale, 2016). Signs of extreme distress, apathy and withdrawal (dissociation) are all adaptations to high levels of dysregulation in a young infant.

Also, very young infants are strongly influenced by their emotional surroundings and seem to sense emotional presence in others and suck it in, experiencing it as their own (Taipale, 2016). If their surroundings are calm and the people around them are calm, the infant also tends to feel calm. Yet, when surrounded by distress, infants tend to catch this mood and feel distressed too. The caregiver's capacity to remain calm and regulated and to keep the infant's environment as calm as possible becomes paramount for the infant's health and well-being, as the caregiver's role is to be a regulatory shield for the infant.

At this Second Level, the infant still needs everything the caregiver gave in the Foundation and First Levels; i.e., to be regulated and responded to through attunement. With good enough parenting, time and repetition, the Second Level is when an infant's sense of self can begin to emerge slowly, and the infant can start the long process of learning to self-regulate.

The Role of Differentiation, Social Recognition and Frustration in Self-Regulation

Meltzoff states that infants, from birth, can recognise others as "like me" (1990) and gain an ability to distinguish others from self relatively early on, perhaps at about 4 to 5 months post-birth. When thinking about differentiation and when this occurs, Taipale points to a quantitative and qualitative distinction of the primary caregiver from other 'others' (2016), and this is perhaps the first indication of some form of differentiation. This differentiation is almost certainly due to the quantity of time the infant spends with the primary caregiver and how both become attuned to each other: "gradually, via repetition, this special influence or relationship qualitatively distinguishes the caregivers' affective presence from the affective presence of other people" (Taipale, 2016, p. 5). By around six months, an infant already seems able to anticipate the caregiver's response due to the consistency of that response to the infant's distress. The infant will adapt their behaviour according to that response (Benoit, 2004) (i.e. the response will be 'organised') and those who feel able to express their negative emotions because they know they will gain comfort and recognition are those infants who are securely attached (van Ijzendoorn et al., 1999).

However, even with poor caregiving, the infant will attach in some way to the caregiver, as humans are genetically programmed to attach as a survival strategy. An infant has absolutely no chance of survival on its own, and so there is no other option but to attach to the caregiver. Infants who are responded to in a consistently negative way will usually develop insecure-avoidant, or insecure-resistant styles of attachment, both of which are still 'organised' because the infant can anticipate the response of the caregiver. In the case of a caregiver who responds in a rejecting or insensitive way, the infant 'avoids' the caregiver and minimises their distress around the parent, hence insecure-avoidant. With a caregiver who is inconsistent, unpredictable or over-involving, the infant will develop an insecure-resistant style. The final style, insecure-disorganised, is a style of attachment that occurs due to exposure to distorted, a-typical and aberrant parenting, which the parent displays not only when the child is distressed, but at other times too. These parents can be dissociated, frightening, sexualised or frightened (Lyons-Ruth, Bronfman & Attwood, 1999). This may be due to the caregiver experiencing unresolved mourning, unresolved trauma (physical or sexual), post-traumatic stress disorder (PTSD) or domestic violence (Zeanah et al., 1999).

When thinking about the stages of infant brain development and how the brain develops, Damon and Hart (1982) recognise the chronological development in infant self-understanding. Rochat (2003) called this "forward engineering" in brain development (p. 117), and it is now known that infants have an implicit representation of self in their social interactions in the first two years of life, but it is not until around two years of age that an explicit self-representation emerges (Kristen-Antonow et al., 2015).

Another development in the infant's brain, at around six months post-birth, is also essential, further underlining the capacity to differentiate between self and other. This is concerning subjectivity. At six months of age, the infant's emotions are no longer totally dependent upon the caregiver's response. Instead, the infant's emotions become more about the caregiver's attitude towards the infant – how they appear, sound, look, and their moods and attitudes, for example – and particularly what the 'other' directs at the infant. This mirroring and how we learn to use others as our 'social mirrors' hugely influence how we feel throughout life. Weinberg et al. (2008) show infant development as beginning with the sensorimotor stage (Piaget, 1952) and also the sensori-affective (Stechler & Latz, 1966) stage, both in infancy. This changes qualitatively as a toddler to incorporate representational and locomotor skills (Piaget, 1962; Beeghly, 1997). Tronick (2007) also added physiologic, behavioural, speech, representational and cognitive components to this developing skill within the infant and called meaning-making systems polymorphic (Weinberg et al., 2008).

A part of the process towards self-regulation comes from the natural diminishment of maternal preoccupation, as life kicks in post-birth, with all the chores and requirements of life and other relationships. The mother can no longer be totally preoccupied with her infant, as this is a fantasy position. This slow reduction in preoccupation leads at the same time to a slowly increasing level of frustration in the infant. Donald Winnicott wrote about infant frustration in 1971 and how important small amounts of frustration are in the infant's growing capacity to differentiate between reality and fantasy and in their ability to tolerate such frustration. Due to years of research on infant development, the Center on the Developing Child at Harvard University also advocates an infant experiencing small amounts of frustration (within reason) as hugely important for an infant's development and their ability to learn to tolerate frustration. A mark of the infant's increasing ability for self-regulation would be a shift from requiring the caregiver to actively assist in their regulation, through rocking, soothing, etc. to helping the infant manage their self-regulation.

The Still Face Experiment video (Tronick et al., 1978) is a prime example of this and allows us to see how an infant of around six to nine months in age can differentiate between what Reddy and Trevarthen (2004) call "engaged" versus "non-engaged" interaction. In the video, the infant is expecting the mother to interact normally with her, but the mother suddenly withdraws all the normal regulatory processes of engagement and mirroring for a matter of around a minute or so. This video shows how quickly an infant becomes dysregulated, in only a matter of seconds, when the caregiver is not mirroring, echoing or attuning to them and seems disengaged with the infant's desire for connection. We can also see how active the infant is in trying to regain connection with the caregiver, taking it upon themselves to articulate and gesticulate their fear and desperation. If the infant constantly has a withdrawn caregiver, it is easy to see why the infant might give up on being active in social interaction and instead withdraw into apathy. Research shows how sensitive children are toward social mirroring and how they use their entire social world to understand who they are (Kristen-Antonow et al., 2015; Rochat, 2009).

This is vital knowledge for therapists working in the perinatal field. The therapist can use it to help parents by offering information and encouragement with this vital parent–infant connection. The parents may not understand the importance or how to provide this connection. Working with mothers and their infants offers a chance for the therapist to show how this connection can happen in real-time. If the mother is experiencing severe depression or is withdrawn, and perhaps is struggling to bond with her infant, this can be deeply shaming, and bring high levels of guilt. However, it is possible to reassure parents that the partner or possibly another close family member can step into this connective void in the short term, so that the mother can gain the help she needs, lessening or eliminating any detrimental impact on the infant's brain and social development. This may go part way to reducing the horrible experience of mother guilt.

It is important to acknowledge that humans are meaning-makers, as Tronick and Bruner (Bruner, 1990) attested, and this meaning-making begins through our relational connection with others. Humans are social creatures and do not develop in a vacuum. An infant begins to form their sense of self only in relation to others and to the environment around them, slowly becoming able to make meaning out of this. Thus, a child experiencing emotional and physical neglect, with an under-stimulating environment, with few toys and little human interaction, will struggle to develop normally, may have delayed speech, cognition and emotional development delays and difficulty with locomotor skills. They might also have difficulty forming a sense of who they are, due to the lack of mirroring and attunement. In extreme examples, the infant's brain development may become stunted or damaged.

When a caregiver is engaged with their infant, the fact that the caregiver shows in their expression and in their behaviour that the infant is 'seen' and also 'heard', fulfils the infant's hunger for recognition. An infant signals their emotion within their entire body, and the capacity for the caregiver to reflect back this emotion, in tone, expression and in visible gestures, is crucial. Again, over time and through repetition, the infant can begin to differentiate between the elements of engagement, such as mirroring and attunement, and non-engagement such as a dispassionate or withdrawn mother. The Child Development Centre at Harvard calls this engagement system between infant and caregiver 'serve and return'. As shown in Figure 6.1, I call it the need and response cycle.

The differentiation between engaged and non-engaged responses also serves us through to adulthood. The ability to "decouple" (Gergely & Watson, 1996, p. 1198) what is our own feeling from that which is clearly the other's is a point of brain development in infancy. The 'mirroring other' provides a form of feedback loop, the caregiver eventually seeming to instinctively 'know' what their infant wants through attunement and attending to their needs. Over time, and with a great deal of repetition from the attuned caregiver, the infant begins to learn to differentiate their feelings, monitor them, reflect on them and distinguish between them, which is a huge step towards self-regulation. The analogy given by Taipale to clarify this is:

> In adult life, consider looking at a mirror and realizing that you look tired; consider, moreover, that you had not explicitly categorized your feeling as tiredness, even if you felt tired already; now, looking at a mirror, you see how tired you look, and this makes you realize that you indeed are tired.
>
> (2016)

All these relational and affective patterns are processed through the infant's amygdala, then encoded and stored. As the infant's hippocampus is not yet properly developed, any critical emotional memories are outside of and beyond conscious awareness, locked away within the amygdala. What is stored are the sensorimotor patterns or schemas, and even body postures, which are often non-narratable and may be felt extremely intensely within the body. Cornell and Landaiche drew our attention to these original intense experiences (2006), and it is on top of these original experiences that our transferential processes (impasses, projective identification, parallel processes, and enactments) sit. Cornell and Landaiche state that when these original intense experiences are touched, which usually occurs within our most intimate relationships, it can trigger a powerful and most intense feeling of both extreme dread and hope, bringing intense anxiety and sometimes despair that may seem intolerable and unresolvable (2006). The birth of an infant is one such moment that can arouse parental protocol, due to the tremendous, unpredictable and unknown elements within this process.

It is also these relational, affective, original, intense experiences and the patterns they form that are the basis of our life positions (Berne, 1976/1962), and this may explain why it is so difficult to change them. Of course, it is also important to acknowledge that these encoded experiences can be positive and negative, not simply pathological. Yet, they do have the capacity to interfere with the infant's relational abilities.

95

Psychotherapy with the Infant in the Room

Working with the mother and the infant in the room may be controversial for some therapists. For example, it could be argued that working with grief and trauma is not ethical in pregnancy. The contra argument to this could be the ethics of not working with this before the birth of the baby, for the sake of the mother–infant fundamental relationship post-birth. I do this type of work with much thought, discussion with the parent, and a great deal of supervision to bring to light the dilemmas posed by the work. Such thought and discussion need to continue throughout therapy so that all parties continue to be comfortable working this way. However, this real-time therapy with the mother–infant bonding and attachment gives an opportunity to shed light on all sorts of things that may sit underneath the disturbance. I look for any clues in this relationship and what they might tell me. Below are a few examples from mothers who sought therapy post-birth.

Mothers with catastrophic thoughts of finding their infant dead or who are fearful of losing them in some way may carry historic unresolved grief from losing a parent or partner or may have been separated from their parents at a young age (going to boarding school at a very young age, for example). It may be difficult for the mother to see any connection to grief, particularly if the loss was unspoken throughout childhood, or the separation was discounted by others in the family. In some families, grief is too huge to process, particularly when combined with a lack of ability to self-regulate. This might mean that a parent who has died is not spoken about and becomes a taboo subject. This type of unconscious, unresolved grief and the subsequent fear of further loss can bring a need to protect the infant from harm and may lead to engulfing, smothering mothering. Perhaps the mother finds it difficult to put her infant down, or to leave the infant sleeping, continuously checking the infant is still alive, or fussing over every small detail in her infant's life. Clues in therapy to this grief changing in the mother would be her choice to leave the infant safely at home with her partner, something that needs to be totally her choice, and not part of the therapist's agenda.

Mothers with twins can, amongst other things, struggle with their relationship with one of their twins. Many things might hamper this. For example, there could be a schism in her relationship with one infant. Perhaps one twin was born naturally, and the second was born by C-section because the mother was too exhausted, forming a gap in her memory and 'knowledge' of her second infant as she has no memory of their birth. It might be that one infant is unwell at birth and needs some extra care in a neonatal special care unit, yet the other infant does not. This may bring anxiety that the mother is not as attached to the poorly infant. Equally, she may favour the poorly infant and give them much more attention. Either way, this can be hugely anxiety-provoking and cause a great deal of inner turmoil and self-criticism. Working with the mother together with her twins may help to reality check her relationship with them both and is an opportunity to feedback my observations.

I see many mothers who struggle with perfectionism in themselves and their infants. Often these are mothers who hold professional jobs requiring a great deal of organisation and meticulousness in their role, and consequently believe they can control every aspect of their pregnancy, birth and the life of their infant. The reality that they cannot, can come as a huge shock. More than this, when parents struggle with relating to their infants, it is possible to help them understand the cues their infant is offering. One mother was convinced her infant "hated" her, because the infant turned her head away from her every time the mother tried to connect with her. Being able to help the mother understand that her infant was a little overwhelmed by her gaze and working with the mother and the infant to change the way she related to her daughter helped to reduce the mother's paranoia, and this then unlocked historic trauma from her own experience of an engulfing mother.

By now, I hope it is becoming crystal clear that neurobiological research into infant development shows just how much time infant development requires, and that it is a long, sequential and repetitive process. Research also shows how much of our early childhood developmental experiences remain with us throughout our lifetime. I would therefore like to offer some reassurance for the many parents who might now be cringing at and feeling hopelessly guilty about the memory of those times when they missed their children through lack of attunement. This requirement for a great deal of repetition in child development means that good enough really is what it means – 'good enough'. The requirement for repetition when giving perinatal psychotherapy is also a necessary factor as it is this repetition that helps to model and solidify the knowledge and experience the client is receiving. Also, as already stated, some small level of frustration is helpful and part of a normal developmental process (for infants and adults). For those parents who had abusive, neglectful and traumatic childhoods themselves, they have what I think of as a void of knowledge. I very much believe that many of these parents, if they had known the importance of connection and self-regulation and had an opportunity in therapy to develop these skills, would have done so. Once they learn about these missing skills, many of the parents I see can gain them in adulthood and this goes a huge way to forming good enough connections with their children.

According to the Center on the Developing Child, the single most common factor for a child to develop resilience and the ability to overcome hardship, is to have at least one person who offers a stable, committed and supportive relationship which

> provides the personalized responsiveness, scaffolding, and protection that buffer children from development disruption. They also build key capacities – such as the ability to plan, monitor, and regulate behaviour – that enable children to respond adaptively to adversity

and thrive. This combination of supportive relationships, adaptive skill-building, and positive experiences is the foundation of resilience.
(Center on the Developing Child, n.d. – Key Concepts)

This person may not be a primary caregiver, but could also be a grandparent, a teacher, a family friend, or a neighbour, if they have a good deal of input with the child growing up.

Finally, I hope it is also possible to see a certain accuracy in Levin-Landheer's theory on cycles of development (1982), as she recognised that these crucial developmental stages in infancy and childhood form a set of building blocks for the next important stages of development to grow upon and she too saw that these developmental stages continue all the way through to adulthood. When one of these building blocks is out of alignment, due to early and continued misattunement, trauma or neglect, it makes it difficult for the infant to have a metaphorical stable surface onto which they can build their next developmental stage. This brings to mind Berne's stack of pennies (1961) being at risk of toppling when warped coins (childhood trauma) exist within the stack. A discussion about whether or not humans do or do not 'recycle' these stages, as Levin-Landheer believed, is unfortunately outside the scope of this book.

In writing this chapter, I realise that some of what I have written might go towards a depth exploration of ego states and how and when they develop in infancy and may be able, at some level, to show how mentalization and Scilligo's model of the structural analysis of social behaviour (2011) may be interlinked. However, although this is an aspect of TA theory which I feel could benefit from such an integration and interlinking, again this is not the place or space in which to do it.

7

1001 WAYS TO DEVISE
A TREATMENT

Treatment Planning

With dialogue from the TA members of Our Evolution:
Sarah Crowley, Valeria Villa, Amy Lennox, Susanne Fuller,
Isa Delannoy, Mihaela-Leocadia Hartescu, Barbara Rupar,
Henrietta Whitfield, Oliver Hunt

This chapter has been a collaborative process with the TA psychotherapy members of a cross-European perinatal group called Our Evolution, which I began in July 2021. I chose to write the chapter in collaboration, firstly, as a support and secondly, because I believe there are many ways to plan treatment, and the members of this group show their creative and flexible thinking about and approaches to working with maternal and perinatal clients. The group met twice to discuss our thoughts and processes around treatment planning. This chapter integrates parts of these discussions with my thoughts and narrative. All dialogue from the group meetings is shown with the speaker's name. When using the 'I' in this chapter, it refers to Emma. When using the 'we', it refers to all the TA members of the group stated at the beginning of the chapter. The members of Our Evolution are cross-cultural, cross-gender, cross-modality and cross-border (country) too. Transactional Analyst members are a group of English, American, French, Romanian, Slovenian and Italian psychotherapists, many of whom are working in a country (England, France, Switzerland, Spain, Slovenia and Italy) and a culture that is not necessarily their own. This diversity gives a richness of knowledge and depth to our experience.

This chapter explores the value and critique of the TA concept of treatment planning, during which we (all of those named above) ask what its purpose is and, more importantly, its usefulness when working with clients experiencing maternal disturbance and distress. As a group, we acknowledge the importance and purpose of a plan and how this can offer a container of safety and security and be a metaphorical 'map' for both therapist and client. We also highlight why work in the maternal sphere may challenge some of the tenets of TA, particularly change and autonomy.

DOI: 10.4324/9781003365822-7

Together, we discussed the differences between working with clients in this transitional period and working with other client presentations. Is it different, and if so, then why? In particular, the levels of parallel process inherent within parenting and therapy are highlighted and the effect these parallels can have within the therapeutic space, which do not necessarily occur when working with other client presentations.

Finally, the aim of this chapter is to open dialogue on treatment planning by questioning its purpose and offering some alternative thinking. Many questions surfaced within the writing process, such as: is treatment planning valuable? Is it useful in its current context in TA at present? Can treatment planning be less formulaic, less rigid, and less contrived? Do we even need a treatment plan? What might we use instead of this formula? What role does this plan play, and most importantly, who benefits from it? There are not necessarily complete answers given to these questions. It is more about opening up and exploring why treatment planning is such a fundamental part of TA and why it is required knowledge for Certified Transactional Analyst (CTA) exams, and challenging what may be seen as the status quo, particularly in training and examining.

Working in the maternal is evolutionary and developmental, which is "the birth of the new, and the rebirth, regeneration and recycling [of the mother]" (Haynes, 2023). The process of bringing a baby into the world is utterly transformative. "And with each story, we change. The therapist changes with each client, so the parent changes with each child" (Isa Delannoy).

Creativity and flexibility are essential when working with this client group due to the intrinsic individuality in the work. There is no 'one size fits all' approach, much like there is no one type of pregnancy, no one type of birth, and no one parenting experience. Clients are so used to being compared to the norm, whatever that is, by medical practitioners, society, family, and friends that it is easy to forget that they are unique.

Every client will bring different stories and experiences as well as symptoms. Each client may also require a different process in treatment. Even if parents have more than one child, each pregnancy will be different, as every child is different, every human is different, and our DNA is different. I want to honour this difference, this individuality; to acknowledge that each of us is unique, and this uniqueness is inherent within the process of conception and birth too. This specificity needs to be accounted for within treatment planning processes.

In the meetings Our Evolution had, there was no right or wrong, no absolute, no 'stage' in mind. For one of us, the most essential thing was holding; for another, it was demystification, or perhaps storytelling or mourning. In all our discussions, the group paralleled something about parenting, each one of us doing it differently, with our client at the forefront, yet with a willingness to listen to other perspectives and to be impacted and shaped by them.

Some Difficulties with the Concept of Treatment Planning

Treatment planning can be daunting for students. Working with exam prep trainees focusing on writing the CTA exam, I have found these two words often bring a negative response from them. It seems common to imagine that the process needs to be linear and forward-looking, which some may imagine is planned early in the work. When there is the realisation that it is not necessarily either of these, some trainees struggle with the concept and perhaps even dismiss it. I wonder if this may be around language – the words 'treatment' and 'planning' can be assumed to be forward-moving processes. Yet treatment planning is often backwards-looking – "Ah, this is what I did, and this is the treatment plan my work fitted into ...".

Sarah Crowley named this difficulty at the start of our first group meeting:

> I have a reaction to the words 'treatment planning' as they are pathologising and move away from the equality/relational stance. I prefer to use 'therapeutic planning' to meet my client wherever she is.

Oliver Hunt also named some of his difficulties:

> [There is] that sort of ambiguity around the concept of treatment planning as something being 'done to' clients. But in the perinatal world, when people come in feeling really dysregulated, [we need to] try to find enough of a process to go "ok what do we need to do first?"

The idea of this 'plan' may seem constricting, rigid, boundaried, inflexible and pathologising to some. Trainees can get stuck with treatment planning, thinking it is outdated, part of the sixties' American pop psychology, medicalising and unhelpful, and something they might only do to pass essays and CTA exams. Indeed, when offering training across-modalities, participants who are not TA trained are often horrified by the concept and cannot understand why TA would still insist on such a thing. So, perhaps my first question is what is the real purpose of a treatment plan, what is it actually for, and more importantly, who does it serve? Isa Delannoy:

> That is a key question. Who do we want to make the treatment plan for? If we don't know why we are doing it, it won't work; it is bound to fail.

In writing this chapter, there felt a critical need to question treatment planning, evaluate its purpose, and confront why it is still considered vital in the TA community. Isa again:

> How important it is to you to feel legitimate in your work. Everyone is different. For some, it [treatment planning] is an obstacle rather than

a support. Being with, the connection, the trust, this is enough to help people realise they can manage, they can cope with the situation. It [parenting] has been done before, and it will still be done afterwards.

From early on in our discussions, nature and the idea of providing a 'map' were central metaphors in our conversation. Sarah:

> Not giving treatment planning any thought would be like a guide offering to lead a hike but turning up without a map and disinterested in what their client wants to see. A treatment plan is like a map. We might get lost; we might backtrack a bit because we saw something we liked in the woods. It is a navigation tool for the therapeutic journey; it supports me, but the term treatment planning, yuk. It needs re-branding.

I quite like the idea of a 'map' with all its possibilities. We (client and therapist) might together choose a pathway, taking one particular direction out of multiple ways we could choose to go. We might deviate from the path; we might even deviate from the map; we might get lost and yet somehow find ourselves back on track again. This possibility of deviation offers me a sense of freedom when thinking about treatment planning, which I believe is much needed due to the uniqueness of the client in front of me. I struggle with a formula for the 'treatment'. My experience of the therapeutic process is that it is non-linear and can go backwards and forwards or even round and round. It cannot be boxed up into stages, and we (my client and I) might need to stay in one place only. All of these differences offer value to the client.

And here is the dichotomy. Some therapists may need a 'container' to hold their clients, and for their clients to feel held, yet they perhaps don't want to feel boxed or hemmed in, nor for their clients to feel like that either. Many of the group certainly did not want to align themselves to a prescribed set of stages or tasks that someone else had written.

Valeria Villa:

> When we treatment plan in TA, we expect the work to progress towards something, when it doesn't. There is a progression, but not in that exact way. Even if we return to the same point, we go in circles; it is so messy. Treatment planning doesn't speak to me. I use the metaphor of the 'post-it' note with clients. Can we put down some words, some things, and some names that we might encounter on the treatment journey? Because Post-it notes can be removed, you can also add more. I don't want to be defined by stages in the journey, so we might skip some. But the note itself does help. It gives freedom not to speak to a stage because we are *supposed* to. We know from the beginning that we can put everything in the mix, but we need to create meaning; the idea that there is a treatment plan and stages feels too artificial to me.

Valeria is speaking of an ongoing group discussion about working to a prescription or a protocol. Maternal work does not fit protocols, probably due again to the specificity of the client. Amy Lennox:

> Rigidity doesn't make sense. We are talking about connecting with intuition and yet [according to Berne] you have got to do it within this plan – how can you take that mass of humanity and put it into a schedule? Flexible structure can be supportive and underpin safety, especially around the client's readiness and availability to go deeper.

Our conversations also picked up on the inherent patriarchy within this terminology – treatment planning. The group has a heightened sensitivity and can sniff out patriarchy in a flash, probably due to high levels of oppression within perinatal work and the maternal space. Why is treatment planning insisted upon? Are we (TA clinicians) only doing it because someone (a man perhaps? Berne himself?) somewhere, back in the 1960s and 1970s, decided this was what was needed to become a Transactional Analyst – regardless of field? This parallels the patriarchy in birth itself, which became entrenched when doctors (on the whole male doctors) began the medicalisation of childbirth. Is TA practice being boxed in by this theoretical medical concept called treatment planning? Where is the diversity? How do we account for intersectionality within what seems to be a prescribed set of 'stages'?

It might also be considered ironic that Berne's writing was of an essential repudiation of the medical model of treatment. Yet, there is a flavour of the medicalisation of the client by insisting on a treatment plan. Berne desired to bring the patient fully into the discussions around their treatment, intentionally using non-medical language, which was simple and understandable for the client, with bilateral contracting to bring transparency to the process. Yet this is simultaneously juxtaposed with the use of a medical model called treatment planning, which may implicitly pathologize the client, implying something is wrong with or perhaps not quite right with the client.

For me, there is also an inherent perception within the word 'planning' of a need to have forward movement (change) in the work and in the client. Something that TA seems to prescribe to within all its theories. However, this medicalisation and need for change does not sit comfortably nor fit with work in the perinatal period, as a therapist may be supporting the client through such elements as normalisation or toleration of a challenging yet normal and natural transitional process. This may challenge the concept of change, with little or no forward movement, bringing to light a consideration about what the word change means.

I often reflect on the medicalisation of conception and birth and the move from normal and natural to medical and artificial. A shift from embracing the multiple different ways to give birth and shoe-horning women into an imposed delivery, laid down, with monitors and drips attached, using instruments many of which were designed in the 17th century, benefitting the medical practitioners rather than the mother and partner; unable and unwilling perhaps to embrace the natural, the difference and the diversity? For me, treatment planning is imbued with power and privilege – a one-up position that situates the therapist as the expert, the one who 'knows' what the process will be, which I find distinctly uncomfortable.

My sense of treatment planning is that it can feel like we are trying to fit a square peg into a round hole, and that treatment planning seems to have little correlation to the perinatal experience. Again, my question remains: who does this serve – the client or the therapist?

Barbara Rupar:

> I work so intuitively, so thinking about treatment planning or the phases within, it almost doesn't feel safe for me. Embodying safety and presence is crucial. I can see the value in planning; I am not opposed to it or discounting it totally. I would very much like to have a map, but as it is, it doesn't really connect with what is present [in perinatal psychotherapy]. It feels like this is a parallel process. There is no one map to matrescence either. A lot of it is intuition, and it's messy sometimes, happening all at once.

Valeria:

> This connects with pain and pleasure in parenting. How can we [therapists and parents] get away from the pain? We know it is painful, but how can we escape the pain? Are mothers/parents happy? Not asking, "Do you have pain?" asking, "Do you have pleasure?"

Perhaps, Valeria and Barbara are voicing how transactional analysts can progress from the prescription that is treatment planning into something more freeing. We know that we need something (a plan, a map?). How can we redefine this to include and encompass all the individuality, uniqueness and difference that our clients come with and focus our clients towards the pleasure of their life?

I think of my work as supporting the client on their journey. They will take me on their journey, and I will walk alongside them. They will forge the pathway. Isa again:

> It is the same as parenting and mentoring. The person who is accompanying is grounded. We know what we know, but there is also a lot that we don't know we know. And our clients will take from us whatever they need, and we can observe the outcome and how things are changing.

In response to Isa, Amy:

> When I go back to the container idea, that is what roots me, the checking in [with my client]. It is not me doing it for them or planning it out. It is rather "Where are you?" "Where do you want to go?" and "What has changed?"

Valeria:

> It is as if in order to have a treatment, we need to have a plan. So, in order to have value in the therapeutic journey, it has to be planned. Yet it doesn't have to be planned; it can just happen."

How do we, as therapists, hold this tension between treatment planning being an important part of TA but that it might not fit comfortably with our work? As Amy notes:

> Treatment planning is a legacy. This is how you do TA, and these are your steps. And that is appealing to me. Is our approach and comfort with treatment planning linked to our script and our defences? Treatment planning helps me feel I am safe enough and confident enough to navigate the road ahead."

In response to Amy, Henrietta Whitfield picks up on another parallel process:

> There is something about the parent being regulated and the therapist needing [also] to be regulated. If they [parents] are not regulated, they are no use to the child. If that is within a treatment plan, then it is important you are in one, and it is the therapist's job to know that, to use or not to use a treatment plan.

Valeria again:

> Treatment planning guides the work, and we also need to step into this stage of life with our clients, not to create something that is different from where they are at.

Are Perinatal Clients Genuinely Different from Any Other Client?

One of the essential discussions the group had was around the difference between working with perinatal clients and working with other client presentations and the importance of this for treatment planning.

One of the first differences we all spoke about was the intense dysregulation that perinatal clients often come with initially. Yes, many clients are dysregulated. The difference may be the intensity of the dysregulation, the impact this has on the client, and the fear of the effect on the infant. Addressing this intense dysregulation forms one of the most critical parts early in the work.

Another essential element is that we are not working with only one client. There is always more than one, even if that 'more than' is a fantasy of a baby that might be. The mother may be pregnant, and what then? Do we stop the depth of the work because of this? Is it ethical to work with a pregnant woman? Is it ethical to steer a pregnant woman away from the work because we might be fearful of what this might do to the fetus when this might offer an opportunity to explore something which unlocks something in her own parenting? Which is better for the client? This work brings many ethical complexities, sometimes even before the work has begun.

Script and Ego State Changes

One ongoing conversation within our group is the sense that giving birth/ parenting is such a fundamental life transition that there is likely to be a shift in script. Becoming a parent changes a person physically, psychologically, physiologically and emotionally from conception. There is a radical change in the mother's hormones, such as progesterone and oestrogen, and some hormones become active and are only present during pregnancy (human chorionic gonadotropin hormone and human placental lactogen). Susanne Fuller:

> If the baby is in the womb, the mother has to metaphorically and physically 'grow' around the fetus and has to metaphorically integrate the infant. It is such a huge change – it is 24/7, and she cannot ever give this infant back. The reality of this is huge and is what mothers come with.

The father's hormones also change at conception, particularly testosterone and estradiol, which I speak more about in Chapter 11 on fathers and partners. Recent research shows these changes in the father enable him to be more supportive and focused towards his partner (Edelstein et al., 2015, 2017; Gettler et al., 2011) rather than focused outside the partnership, looking for another mate. There are risks to human survival if the father is not focused on and protective of the mother and infant, with the possibility of her being left high and dry trying to support and provide for her infant alone.

What happens to our script when this realisation hits us? How does this transition in responsibility from being someone's child to becoming someone's parent push against or challenge script? It will impact it somehow. The perception we hold of ourselves will be challenged, provoked, questioned, tested even and may fundamentally shift. Is this why so many mothers and fathers talk about feeling they have lost who they are or have lost a sense of self? In TA, the transition and script shift occurring within adolescence has already been highlighted. There is also an acknowledgement that changing careers can be life-altering. Becoming a parent is another time ripe for a fundamental shift in script.

I have been curious for a long time about what happens in our ego states during this period.

Henrietta:

> In some way, the mother is born again as an adult. Things like injunctions or script messages are perhaps completely different before matrescence [the process of becoming a mother]. It is almost like there is an entirely new script, a new everything; they [mothers] come into their body for a second time. There is a level of awareness of an adult having lived a life, but there is also an unawareness, a newness and a lack of symbolisation in what is now. Almost like being a child in an adult's body, like landing on an alien planet, where although you have all of your capacities, you are also completely new, paralysed in the birth of the baby, with a lack of symbolisation. Like the mother has no map, there are no markers for this, and a new language needs to be learned.

Sarah, in response to Henrietta:

> Or she has the cultural symbolisation, which leaves her adrift because there is a stereotypical "how happy, how perfect and wonderful" it is going to be.

Susanne:

> And the cultural difference in that perhaps having a baby in Spain or Italy is very different to China or Britain.

I hear this discombobulation, this feeling like a child in an adult's body, a great deal in my client work. I have clients who struggle with this as parents, and we often explore this sense, which I call 'Adulting'; this tension between feeling like they are not a grown-up and yet knowing they are a parent and therefore 'should' feel grown up. How can you be a grown-up but not a grown-up? It feels like a myth that, somehow, we grow up when we have children. We can be thrust into adulthood, but there can be a dissonance, thrust into it but unable to meet it, a gap between these two.

Thinking about giving birth in terms of TA, something may shift and change in both our script and our ego states. Before becoming a parent, the Parent ego state is filled with parental introjects from other parents or parental figures. When we become a parent, we have a different sense of ourselves as a parent, and maybe there is a shift in our Parent ego state, or perhaps we hold a new Parent in our Adult. Oliver:

> Thinking about the one or three ego state models, if Parent and Child are purely historical, then the new parental functioning happens in Adult because it is a response to the here and now, rather than being historical. There will be times when we respond from our Parent rather than our Adult. Almost like there is this potential for a new part of us to grow and emerge in Adult.

Susanne:

> Thinking about it in relation to the integrating Adult model, perhaps instead of integrating split-off parts, we are bringing something new, incorporating something new, which is a script shift.

I think we are bringing something new. We think we know who we are going to be as a parent, but actually, we don't have a clue until we are indeed through the birth process and find ourselves with our newborn infant absolutely and utterly reliant on us for everything that infant needs. It can feel wonderful and utterly terrifying at the same time. The birth of the infant and the birth of the parent. A new role we have never had before and could not have quite imagined how it might be.

Different Therapeutic Planning Processes

To honour the differences within the group, I have first given my thoughts on how I envisage what may occur within the treatment, then given brief descriptions of other elements group members spoke about in our discussions. Table 7.1 shows the elements I think about when working in the maternal/perinatal sphere. Rather than use the word 'stages', I use the terms elements and experiences instead. The transition into parenthood is suffused with feelings and experience, and calling these 'stages' fits, yet does not fit at all, so I prefer to use elements and experiences as they feel more congruent to what I am showing.

I have diagrammed these elements previously in the shape of a triangle (Haynes, 2022a), and this is how I feel they are best represented, each element building on the one below, not ever separate processes, more an expanding, developmental, evolutionary process. What I believe is important is that the infant is held in focus through the parent during treatment. Thus, I have chosen to show the three elements together in column form – client (parent), therapist and infant. There is something so familiar when a client arrives in crisis, often deeply distressed and sobbing, that parallels something of the newly born distressed infant. I recognise this as the client recycling their early infancy stage, confused and mystified by this world, with sudden, intensely disturbing feelings which need to be immediately recognised and removed by the '(m)-other'. In this state, an infant has no way to release their feelings, so

Table 7.1 Treatment Stages in Perinatal Psychotherapy Using the Developmental Stage in the Client and Their Therapeutic Requirement and How These Relate to Infant Development

Client	Therapist	Infant Development
Crisis	*Attune to*	*Birth*
helpless		helpless
loss of/no sense of self	Crisis management. Attune and respond to client's distress and basic needs, provide safety and security, information seeking, primary contracting	Reflex stage – Pain (cries), no pain (sleep)
Little or no self-regulation		No self-regulation
Need & Response cycle active		Need – Response cycle begins
Mystification – who am I?		**Basic need**: to be cared for, recognition hunger – carer to regulate infant to remove pain/distress (food, warmth, safety, touch)
Colonised by the infant (or fantasies of the infant)	Help client to find language for storytelling	
Basic need: therapist to recognise me and attune to help remove pain/distress	Begin to demystify client's process	
To feel safe and secure	Attuning to client's Child	
To begin to narrate story		
Connection	*Connection*	*Connection*
Self to 'other'		(week 8/9 onwards)
Forming the therapeutic alliance/relationship	Forming attachment	Seeks out relationship, smiles, eyes begin to focus, responds to the 'other', Need – response cycle
Need/response cycle	Respond to the client's cycle	
Basic need: To have a therapeutic alliance/relationship with therapist, to feel attuned and respond to, therapist to repair any ruptures	misattunement/attunement, re-contracting, deepening therapeutic alliance	**Basic need**: 'other' to regulate affect and to be responded to through attunement
	Listening to client's Child and new Parent ego state	
Integration	*Constant Object*	*Attachment*
Gaining a new sense of self		(begins from 4–6 months)
Learning who I am now (new Parent and Adult ego states forming)	Be a constant object	Reaches out for contact sense of self begins emerging
	Help to regulate affect	
Grief for loss of who I was before	Respond through attunement, moving into the intrapsychic space	**Added need**: Object Constancy, response from 'other' becomes critical
Heading towards health and Individuation	Mourning versus pleasure	
	Strengthening new Adult	

these can escalate quickly into a state of extreme distress as if they might be dying. For the client, there can be severe anxiety and fear, which they mask until they are in crisis and can no longer mask these intense feelings.

The Possible 'Stages' of Treatment

Crisis Management

I think about treatment planning firstly as attending to the crisis the client comes with. This is because in perinatal work the client is often in crisis, and typically there is a heightened state of dysregulation and trauma, possibly because the client has been in a high level of crisis for an extended period of time. If this crisis is not addressed, the dysregulation prohibits cognition, and there is often little Adult ego state to work with. How do I soothe the Child ego state enough to begin to form an empathic bond with my client? How do I make it safe and secure enough for them to share their story with me and initiate a connection that can lead to the therapeutic alliance?

An intensely dysregulated parent cannot remain calm and cognitive (in Adult), working with their infant to regulate/co-regulate them. Infant regulation is such a fundamental part of the parenting role that I know I need to help the parent to a calmer place so that they, in turn, can calm their infant. In the first weeks of life, the infant has no capacity at all for any form of regulation and is 100% reliant on the parent/caregiver to regulate them. Over time, and with good enough care, this will move slowly towards co-regulation, with the parent calming the infant and also modelling calm so that the infant can begin to learn to regulate itself. However, the difficulties and stressors of modern life are such that many of my clients have never learnt how to do this for themselves and say they have lived in constant anxiety or stress. Modelling and then teaching clients how to do this can be fruitful for the sake of everyone in the family.

When we explored this first aspect of therapy, group members had similar and yet different thoughts on this aspect. Valeria:

> At the beginning, with couples or parents, there is a lot around needs, which don't emerge in the same way with other clients.

Amy agreed:

> It is more about hearing and holding, helping affect regulation, building the empathic bond and the therapeutic alliance before I can get to decontamination, or strengthening the Adult.

This Amy called "setting the container". Barbara:

> Dysregulation is often on another level to other clients. For me, there is something about safety and the injunctions around it – "Don't feel

safe". Through establishing safety, deepening the empathic bond, as Amy said, and through modelling the internal structure, deconfusion is already happening from the beginning ... The therapist almost holds the client's internal Child, nurturing, soothing and normalising. I think we provide deconfusion much earlier, by default than other treatment plans.

Storytelling: the Static Space – Colonisation

For Isa, storytelling is a crucial part of the work:

> Listening to their story and whatever it is, normalising it. This can be transformative. If this is what we think of as our task, we make ourselves available as parents, and the child takes what they need.

Henrietta responded to Isa's idea of normalising:

> Normalising the place new mothers find themselves in because there is so little cultural help or cultural conversation about the psychological impact and the early stages.

Returning to the sense of the circularity of the therapeutic process, Valeria spoke of the importance of the "old and the new" in the story and how it is possible to notice this with clients:

> In each of our sessions, what is old at this moment and what is new? That impacts me and the way I think about the client and our relationship in the present and moving forward.

Henrietta:

> I've been struck by thinking there is nothing new in each session, we seem to be in the same place, a static-ness, but it is actually not true; the new is invisible. The mother is so preoccupied that there is a sense of static-ness, and in each session, it feels as if you are going back to the same place. Actually, there is so much going on, but it is not necessarily 'there', not available to the therapist or even the consciousness of the mother. The mother's capacity to engage is a big part of treatment planning.

I'm often thinking about how, with a new mother (not necessarily with a second or subsequent baby), that sense she might have of "I'm here, and nothing seems to change", particularly if the baby has colic, for example. That sense of "this is grinding me down", "I'm not seeing any change", "I don't know what to do", "When will this end". I am wondering if this is another parallel process, that there might not be any visible newness, but just like the infant growing and evolving at a pace that is actually very fast but can appear

111

to a mother to be quick yet terribly slow, particularly if it is a difficult stage. Henrietta picks up this thread:

> What I am thinking about is how the mother's mind becomes completely colonised by the baby. So, the therapist's experience of the mother might be that the mother is static, stuck in one place because they are colonised. But actually, the mother is changing, and a lot is going on. It seems to be static, but it is not.

Emma Haynes:

> And it is all happening, just behind the scenes. It might not be visible, but suddenly the mother is thinking, "Oh", perhaps when she contrasts a nappy from the first days. Then suddenly the nappies seem two or three times the size.

Amy:

> Time is quite a big issue because it contracts and expands, it drags and is speedy, and in thinking about treatment planning, you can try to box it all off in spreadsheet boxes, but it's so amorphous.

Emma:

> Or with a colicky baby, it feels as though it's been forever. This baby won't stop crying, won't sleep, and that sense of "will it ever be any different?"

Barbara agrees:

> The reality of this 24/7 dependency is scary and might feel suffocating, or engulfing. At the same time, feeling "will this ever end, will I ever be separate again?"

Susanne:

> For that reason, the holding is really very important, that weekly space, it can be so comforting, that sense that somebody knows.

Storytelling: Mystification

Amy brought Steiner's concept of demystification and the word colonisation (Minikin & Tudor, 2015) into the discussion and how important normalising the experience is.

> Mystification is about oppression. There is a patriarchal construct [in motherhood] that serves one section of society, and that is built on to

make us accept that it is normal and mothers are abnormal. Mystification infuses beliefs about self, others and the world. This 24/7 care is mystifying; you will have sleep deprivation, and your baby may have colic; rather than it's going to be blissful, it's not going to hurt; your relationship is going to be hunky dory when this new person comes in between you. It's romanticised and demystification is such a big part in this work, whether its infertility, or miscarriage, we are kind of 'set up' that we are going to have this blissful experience and when it doesn't happen it's such a shock.

For Amy, mystification is a big theme for mothers due to the expectation of bliss and immediate competence. In response to Amy, Henrietta:

There is something that is an addition to storytelling. It is important for the mother to narrate for themselves and then for the therapist to bring out the ordinary in it, because a lot is both profound and ordinary, and clients can get stuck in their story in an isolating way, separating from themselves and from community. The demystification is that you are not alone, it's not just you experiencing this at the basic sense.

Mourning versus Pleasure

Henrietta brought up loss within the work we do, which began a conversation around mourning versus pleasure and how much of our work is about grief. Henrietta:

The perinatal has so many losses, the loss of self, the loss of relationship, the loss of identity.

Isa, in response to Henrietta:

Yes there is mourning, there is grieving the loss of lots of things, and there is the rebirth of the person as a parent, the big transition, we have to reconstruct our identity as our child grows inside us and when it is raised. We are changed by the child, in the same way as we are changed by our clients. There is natality for us, not just of the baby.

Within maternal work there can be a fine line between life and death, as the expectations the client holds don't necessarily materialise – pregnancy does not mean an infant is born. This can mean the work feels heavy and overwhelming at times. There is so much that can go right and so much that can equally go wrong, from the disappointment of infertility through to the realisation that parenting is not at all what was perhaps expected. Isa highlights how big this transition into parenthood actually is, and the birth of something new in us, the natality in us and the infant.

With grief and mourning comes the birth of the new, something Valeria is passionate about when working with parents:

> When you named mourning, Henrietta, I thought about how pleasure is important. It's part of perinatal work, is it a moment in treatment planning, how much pleasure is here? Perhaps you so want a child that you structure your life and in that there is death. The two are so connected, something so pleasurable and yet there can be so much grief, loss of the self. Yet there is the element of pleasure in there. Where is the pleasure, where is the fun?

Amy:

> I see that with my couples, where is the fun? You have yearned and yearned for this baby and the capacity for fun has been stripped away, and building that back in.

Barbara:

> Pleasure is part of the injunctions around security, "don't enjoy", "don't feel pleasure". I think it goes hand-in-hand with safety.

Amy:

> I am thinking about cultural injunctions – what if we are mothers who are rolling with this and having too much fun – and I know this is set up, this kind of bliss. But underneath there is a more pernicious message that if you are actually having fun, we cannot possibly have that.

Susanne:

> Sometimes I think that we [therapists] are like trees, when a new branch comes, the shape of the tree changes, and when a branch drops off, the tree can also heal around it and the wood becomes more beautiful. All these things have impacts on us, every client, every stillbirth, every miscarriage, every live birth.

Emma:

> We carry those cells from previous children, and carry those cells from those babies who were stillborn or miscarried, we carry a trace of them, a bit like we carry a trace with us of all our clients.

Short-Term versus Long-Term Work and Timing

In treatment planning, there is a difference in working short term and long term, something the group picked up on. Amy:

> [In long-term work] there is less urgency that we have got to be 'ok enough' in 12 sessions, and I find the context is different. There is something about the nature of the clients coming and the way they come. In 12 sessions, I have to anchor myself, begin looking at ending in session six and that's really only when we are starting to get the empathic bond, when the work is beginning to happen. Whereas in private practice, I can pick and choose more fluidly, there is more space and time to put the jigsaw pieces together and create more of a picture.

Henrietta agrees with Amy:

> In my experience the difference can be the demographic. In charities the clients perhaps don't have social security, don't have the family support, and this is a generalisation. Whereas in private practice the clients can afford to pay for a start, and maybe have more resources and more support. This impacts the treatment planning in terms of how long you have, the context, what you are addressing.

Amy:

> And the people in the charity have often had a longer wait.

Mihaela-Leocadia Hartescu (Leo) adds to this by addressing the differences in seeing clients at pre-conception, pregnancy, and post-birth:

> I'm thinking of the difference of women or parents who arrive in therapy two, three, four years into a child's life where it seems possible for deeper work. They might still be dealing with trauma or are still impacted but are in a different place and different work may be possible. This is different to women in the first weeks and months coming with their baby in the session, because that impacts the session as well. For example, how do you touch on mother rage when the mother is holding her baby and we are online, as opposed to if she can attend by herself, face-to-face and someone else can attend to the baby.

Amy agrees:

> If I am with a mum who is nursing her baby it is different. There is a change in the treatment plan when she has the faith and agency to leave

115

her baby with someone else. I find this is a pivotal moment. It gives me a signal that I can start checking out if we are ready to go deeper.

Henrietta:

> I think it is a parallel process – in the same way the infant is a bit of a barrier between the mother and the therapist, I think the baby is a barrier between the mother and the outside world. As the infant grows, the treatment changes, it grows a little more independence, or the needs become less intense. The mother has more capacity to engage with the treatment. Engagement can mean quite a lot in planning treatment. Any plan has to take maternal preoccupation into account because the mother's capacity to engage in something that isn't the infant is quite minimal.

Conclusion

Much like a birth plan can be useful, a treatment plan also has value as a lightly held guide or map, flexible enough to shift and sway with the multiple experiences of the client. At whatever stage of development the therapist is, trainee, newly qualified, long-standing professional, there is a myriad of ways in which the therapist may choose to 'plan'. For some it may be through words and stories, or it is by using a metaphorical map, for others it might be support through grief and mourning. The 'plan' may be non-linear, circular, unorthodox even, and static. Rather than being reductive, this diversity offers countless opportunities for therapist and client, and opens up the possibility for creative exploration within the therapeutic space.

I find it helpful to hold the developmental stage of client in mind and to draw some parallels from infant development, using this to guide me about what the client may relationally need from me as 'other'. The three levels of development I use: crisis, connection and integration provide a loose metaphorical containment in which the relationship between therapist and client can grow enough so that the therapist can support and sustain the client. This is a parallel process much like the womb being the container for the fetus, supporting, nourishing and sustaining it, allowing the fetus to grow and evolve into whatever form they will be, in order to be 'born' and to individuate.

Who benefits from having a plan – therapist or client? In my mind, the answer may be neither and both. Neither, because some 'plans' or protocols can be held too tightly, rigidly adhered to, structured to suit 'the norm', inflexible and counterintuitive. Such plans or protocols seem to be trying to fit all of humanity into one type, and this is normally due to economic boundaries, i.e., the cost of therapy. I cannot see how this is possible. Humans need to honour the diversity and intersectionality that exists within each of us, and to a treatment plan with the client as the focus, not the plan.

Can relational work in the maternal sphere even be 'planned'? It certainly can be messy and filled with all manner of elements: the 'need and response' cycle, attachment, crisis, and rupture and response when needs are not met. Yet, a plan offers something, a metaphorical first step for the therapist to encourage the client to take towards finding their own pathway to walk along, perhaps. In therapy, it is possible to experience and explore parts together. Maybe it is more helpful to shape treatment planning as a 'whole', just like pregnancy is a whole, offering the container of protection that the client needs in order to grow into their new role. There is also recycling in this, the need or desire for a client to recycle aspects of their development that were lacking, or even missing.

No matter what, our clients seem to find a way through this transition that works for them. We can accompany them on their journey into parenthood, but we cannot tell them how it will be, who they should be, or how to do it. Let's leave Amy to finish off this conclusion with her reflections about TA and what it can offer parents:

> If we are thinking of bringing all the breadth of TA theory into how we each use it differently in treatment planning, it is the permission to be the parent you want to be that honours you and your child. And if you have multiple children each one will be different and will need something different. There is no right or wrong, it's all our unique stories within treatment planning.

8

SPEAKING BEYOND WORDS

Using Creative Methods to Unlock Silence

Creativity is like finding a key to unlock a hidden door into the mother's unknown. What tends to come through the door is what Bollas so beautifully calls the "unthought known". Creative methods allow my client to speak beyond words and bring freshness and unfamiliarity to perinatal psychotherapy. Often, what they unlock is a surprise to both of us. This newness may be new narrative, new responses, new action. Whatever the newness is, perhaps it is a way of speaking the unspeakable, and feeling the un-feelable, permissions that perinatal clients are rarely afforded.

I use creative methods in my perinatal work with clients, supervisees, groups, individuals and couples. I have also used it when training. Creative methods are qualitative research tools used for data collection. Such methods may include visual (photo-elicitation) and narrative (storytelling) techniques. I have written about creativity and creative methods before. I devoted a chapter to creativity in my first book *Motherhood and Mental Illness* (Haynes, 2022b). I have also written an article about creativity for the journal *Transactional Analysis Psychotherapy* (Haynes, 2022a) in which I describe my use of creative objects with perinatal clients. In this chapter I do not want to repeat myself by writing again about creative objects. Instead, I want to add to the theory and describe other creative methods I use, showing some examples possible.

The reason I want to write about creativity and creative methods here is to highlight how they offer possibilities to unlock the silence inherent in the perinatal experience. I don't see creativity or creative methods being used much in TA psychotherapy, yet I find they offer so much possibility. There is a myth that creativity is innate, yet according to research, this is untrue. It is quite possible to learn how to be creative (Csíkszentmihályi, 1990; Scott, Lertiz & Mumford, 2004). Creativity means progress, a vital process in evolving and advancing. It is fostered and developed in a culture of curiosity and exploration. Fear, lack of motivation, grandiosity and the self-preservation drive can easily squash it.

Whenever I talk about using creativity, I am curious to see the response others have to this word. Mostly, their faces light up, and when asked, many say this word offers permission to be child-like and play. Children are usually

DOI: 10.4324/9781003365822-8

free to play, and with this freedom comes imagination and often huge creativity, as they are not yet tied up in rules, regulations and fear of failure. If the person's face doesn't light up, I become curious, wondering what it is about creativity that might feel hampering. Is it scary? Was their creativity squashed at school, so they have lost the knack of using it? What does it mean to express themselves freely? What does it stir up – judgement, ridicule, fear of lack of talent, perhaps?

Creative methods bring something implicit to perinatal psychotherapy. Conception is, in essence, a particular form of creativity that continues in utero. No one knows what their baby will look like, how or who it will be; this is all part of the tension of excitement and fear in pregnancy. The parents can only guess and hope, as well as try desperately to perceive more of their child through ultrasound scans, which many do, of course. However, with the rise in artificial reproductive techniques (ART), the joy and spontaneity of creation and the creativity inherent within it can be sucked away and replaced with never-ending temperature charts, dipsticks, endless monitoring, injections, and the tracking of ovulation dates. These can all too easily become an obsession and fuel anxiety, yet at the same time can be reassuring, a way of taking control of the conception journey.

Creativity is helpful because it can help unlock unconscious processes explicitly and implicitly. On an explicit level, I often use a creative 'object' of my client's choice which they feel describes some part of their perinatal experience or process. This gives us a visual (auditory or spatial) representation of their experience, something we can explore together and co-create meaning from. On an implicit level, using the transferential process can help us to explore the youngest patterns laid down in those first critical 1000 days, the "primary relational patterns" (Cornell & Landaiche, 2006, p. 203), protocol.

In perinatal work, creative methods can be used to unlock both silence and protocol, but also to promote exploration of somatic feeling and implicit cues, to deepen attunement, and enliven a process if it seems stuck or deadened due to an impasse. Implicit cues are the earliest ways humans have been shaped by their environment, influencing how we think, not just what we think (Schwarz & Clore, 2007) and are encoded in our protocol. These can impact us, particularly in states of hyperarousal, when threats can constrict our attention and creativity. Conversely, in positive or 'benign' emotional states, attention and creativity can seem to expand (Friedman & Förster, 2010).

I use creativity to help unblock 'stuckness'. I may have a sense that therapy has stalled, for example, because the client keeps returning to the same topic in a repetitive way. I know there is stuckness when time drags intolerably, I am bored or feel deadened, and there is a chance I will nod off if I don't attend to the process. This sense of stuckness gives me vital clues. It is a time to pay attention to the countertransference, as this may be key information, a crucial strand or detail, locked away or unspoken (a third-degree impasse, perhaps) and inaccessible to the therapeutic process.

Stuckness is a rich source of information that something is blocked, caught or immobile. An unblocking, or a perception of movement, may show change in the psychotherapeutic process, leading to flow (Csíkszentmihályi, 1990, 1996). Flow is so important in psychotherapy. It is a time when the therapist and client are working intuitively and can feel utterly absorbed and immersed in the process, making time fly. Csíkszentmihályi describes flow as follows:

> My mind isn't wandering. I am not thinking of something else. I am totally involved in what I am doing. My body feels good. I don't seem to hear anything. The world seems to be cut off from me. I am less aware of myself and my problems.
>
> (1988, p. 195)

Flow is a time when our bodies are involved at the same time as our minds. In Buddhism and Hindu literature there is a similar something that can be achieved through mindfulness and yoga.

Returning to stuckness, if I have a sense of this in myself or the process, it almost always helps me to think creatively. However, when I *try* to be creative, I often find this is the least creative moment in the therapeutic exchange. Writing this chapter is a case in point. I became bogged down in it, but I was unsure why. What was bogging me down, me the subject, or *trying* too hard? Every time I tried to write my creative thinking became blocked. Stuckness needs a different, unplanned, left-field intervention to transform a block into a flow. What I find essential is that I am using my body so my mind is free.

Maternal disturbance and distress means that women and their infants can become marginalised and lost in a system that seems disinterested in hearing from them. Alienation has been written about at length by Minikin (2011, 2018, 2020, 2021a, 2021b, 2024), and ostensibly, it is alienating for those parents experiencing any form of perinatal disturbance. My question continues to be: how can I facilitate those who feel alienated and silenced, or who silence themselves, to speak up and, more importantly, be heard? I believe creativity and creative methods are useful tools for this process.

Finding My Creativity

My first exploration of the different creative methods available for research helped me understand how important, but also how human creativity is. I gained some understanding that a lack of creativity, or ability to be creative, could offer me essential information about my client's internal process and what might be happening between us in the intersubjective space. Influences on my creative thinking began with an in-depth exploration of the psychoanalytic way of knowing by the mother. This encouraged me to explore the earliest form of knowing, which Ettinger calls "matrixial knowing" (2006, 2010); Lorenzer's "scenic understanding" (1977, 1986); the location of Bion's "origin of knowledge", in reverie, containment and communicative projective identification (1962, 1967); and Winnicott's "transitional space" (1953, 1956/1984, 1960, 1963, 1971/2005). A few of my perinatal clients found creativity difficult, and I became curious about what may have happened and when, to frustrate or block their process. I believe that something can happen in the earliest moments of a person's life when protocol is being formed, and this can stifle creativity. Fear and trauma are other blocks to it, too. I am still exploring so many facets of creativity and the creative process. This is an area which continues to fascinate me and forms a great deal of my research in the maternal.

One path of exploration of elements that hinder creativity fits with my knowledge of the importance of safety and security, encoded in protocol, which I shared in Chapter 5. Is psychological safety and security essential for a person to be creative in psychotherapy? According to Patricia Riddell, Professor of Applied Neuroscience, psychological safety is paramount for creativity, and this was first discovered from research by Kahn (1990). It makes sense that if clients do not feel safe and secure in their therapeutic environment, their creativity will be shut down or hampered, almost certainly due to a lack of cognitive capacity, as they will automatically focus on self-preservation. Thus, safety and security are hugely important in perinatal psychotherapy. However, creativity can also be born out of frustration and need. Certainly, for some perinatal clients, when they are in a crisis position, this can spark immense creativity to free themselves. For others, they remain frozen. What is the difference between these two individuals?

What Is Creativity?

To explain what I mean by creativity I use these words: novelty, effectiveness (Cropley, 2011) and originality (Andreason, 2011), combined with Andreason's quote: "characterised by flashes of insight that arise from unconscious reservoirs of the mind and brain" (2011, p. 42). I feel that the visual form can be "immediate, authentic and offers something the verbal account cannot (Spencer, 2011)" (Haynes, 2022a, p. 135) and can add to the narrative form that is psychotherapy, helping to enrich it. Contextualising creativity in this way allows me to anchor myself and offers me a sense of what might be occurring with my perinatal clients.

Relational TA theory favours creativity because it advocates using all available means (narrative, somatic and visual) to gain information about the client's world, thinking and experiences. When these are woven together with the client's narrative, they form part of the diagnosis. This would include using the transferential domain and visual cues such as movement, gestures and behaviour, which can help us gain a sense of immediacy and authenticity within the therapy. Body movements have already been linked to ego states in TA by David Steere (1981). I would add to this by encouraging the use of reverie, verb sequencing, intuition, symbols, metaphors and paralinguistics.

Paralinguistics are a form of metacommunication that add crucial nuance and depth to the narrative form yet can be overlooked in psychotherapeutic training. The elements included in this 'language' are facial expressions, body language and postural cues, prosody, intonation, volume, tone and pitch of voice. This is precious information which can help guide our perception of our client's world, and the cues from paralinguistics may also be termed "implicit relational knowing" (Lyons-Ruth, 1998). This type of knowing has been defined by Duarte, Martinez and Tomicic as: "the interpersonal knowledge procedurally acquired in relationships with others since the earliest childhood. This knowledge operates outside the attentional focus and the conscious verbal experience of the self (Lyons-Ruth, 1999; Stern et al., 1998)" (2020, p. 440, footnote 1). These implicit cues are so much faster than thinking, analysing, deciding and acting upon (explicit cognitive cues) and form the moments of discordance or synchrony between mother and infant, and are the foundation stones of attachment (Beebe et al., 2010, 2012).

For women and parents experiencing perinatal disturbance (felt within both the body and the mind), creativity and creative methods offer a way to allow their voices (and bodies) to speak louder and beyond the words they utter through whatever medium is used. I can then highlight their 'voices' (both conscious and unconscious) to bring these women in from the margins, which may help towards "reclamation" (Minikin, 2024). My hope, by doing this, is to provide a means of empowerment, to help them feel more in control of what they are experiencing, and to bring some of the unknown out of the shadows and into the light. Those who feel marginalised and alienated are likely to feel out of control, which amplifies anxiety and fear.

Why Creativity?

Berne had a vast creative capacity, which, for TA, began with his interest in intuition (1949). Chiesa has used creativity in TA psychotherapy with children (2012a, 2012b, 2014). Cornell also embodies creativity, which is seen through his writing, particularly in his "Aspiration or Adaptation" article (2010) and his commentary on the writing of Knoblauch (2011), both of which I have highlighted previously. Cornell's article on *Games, Play and Intimacy* (2015), was also helpful to me, as it was an introduction to the work of Cowles-Boyd and Boyd (1980a, 1980b) and helped me to link play and intimacy. I often find that creativity brings more intimacy into the therapeutic relationship, and Cornell's article, although talking about game-playing rather than creativity, seemed to offer me a missing link. I have also already stated that Berne used creativity in his work. There are other writers outside of TA that I have also found useful to explore, such as Milner (1952/1987a, 1952/1987b, 1952/1987c), Ogden (2012), Ritter & Dijksterhuis (2014), and Ritter et al., (2012, 2020), Winnicott (1971). These writers have similarly used creativity as a way to 'unlock' the unconscious.

Returning to Berne and intuition as a form of creative process, how do we build and hone our intuition as psychotherapists, and practitioners? Kottler and Hecker (2002) speak of the centrality of intuition with divergent and convergent thinking in creativity. I often work in the intersubjective space, almost certainly due to the importance of this space in the communication and attunement process for an infant and their mother. Marks-Tarlow speaks of the intersubjective space when she talks about the importance of intuition in therapy:

> Where theory is static, intuition is alive. Where theory exists outside of real time, intuition involves immersion within lived moment. When clinicians become immersed in this fashion, we often attain states of flow (Csíkszentmihályi, 1990, 1996) with our patients. When in a state of flow, therapists get caught up in the throes of implicit processes as intuitively guided.
>
> (Marks-Tarlow, 2018, p. 146)

When thinking about stuckness and passivity in the therapeutic process, perhaps creativity and intuition, combined with divergent and convergent thinking, are the catalysts to the concept of liberation of the mind (Minikin, 2024). Perhaps these are some of the elements in therapy that wake up the sleeping minds of our oppressed, marginalised clients and offer freedom from deception, and an opportunity to awaken our Free Child.

Carson and Becker (2004, p. 111) state that

> creative therapy involves a synergistic combination of the unique personalities involved in therapy, the process of therapy (the way in which change and growth occurs, often involving novel, original or imaginative methods), and the product of therapy (that which is different about people and relationships at the end of therapy).

For Carson and Becker, creativity can be nurtured in both ourselves and our clients, and I think this nurturing could be helpful for those clients who are the most marginalised or oppressed and particularly for perinatal clients.

Using Failure to Promote Reflective Capacity

Creativity fits into evolutionary processes and is developmental, too. Humans grow and develop through evolutionary processes from conception. For example, trial and error, something babies are extremely good at, is about repeated attempts, through backwards reflection, altering what is not working and trying again. Yet many adults seem to think mistakes are wrong and need to be hidden away under the proverbial carpet or denied and discounted. This can lead to a trap of blaming and shaming, a block to the change process, not just in perinatal psychotherapy.

I am interested in how to expand thinking and behaviour for my perinatal clients, and for my working in this field. I want to help them continue to evolve so that they can experience true growth, potential, and physis, rather than get stuck and become immoveable. Creativity can help this. For example, continuing to try is not about throwing the method away because it failed, but learning from mistakes. Yet, to try can have pejorative connotations. The Try Hard driver never came across as something to be encouraged – more to be discouraged when I was training. However, trying over and over is one of the most important abilities a child has in learning and is the difference between mastery and giving up. Mistakes are so valuable as a learning tool for adults, too (see Matthew Syed's book *Black Box Thinking*, 2015) and are to be encouraged as a part of learning. Creativity encourages learning from mistakes, accepting that they happen all the time, and that they are part of an expansive process of discovery.

My learning is definitely hinged on the errors I have made, which have been numerous. I now realise that if creativity does not work with a client, there is usually an excellent reason. In perinatal therapy, a suggestion about using a creative method, a sand tray perhaps, or drawing and playdoh, may be missing the client, refocusing the process forward, when it needs to go backwards and slow down. The suggestion may be discordant with the client's lack of safety within the therapeutic dyad, which can be readily assumed (by the therapist). If I have a sense of discordance, I need to stop and ask myself where my suggestion for creativity has come from. Is it due to my discomfort or fear of failure at that moment? I know I can flounder at the trickiest of moments, weighing up the need to step in to resolve something, or to shift the energy and focus. However, if I can remain reflective of my work and explore what happened, perhaps the reality may be that I was not attuned enough to my client, and I missed them, leading to my client being unable to express themselves or speak out. I have found this to be particularly true when working with clients who have a desire to please me.

This brings me to the word fail. This word has such negative connotations, and I hear it used often by my clients: "I am such a failure as a mother", "I failed giving birth as I had to have a C-section", "my baby fails to thrive". How can this word be reframed positively in the perinatal, but also more widely, as a means for learning, innovation and growth, helping us develop, rather than something to shy away from and try and ignore? I like to think that if I bring my own creativity into the therapeutic space, perhaps I can enable my client to find their creative ability too, to help shift the power towards them and the resources they thought they did not have, and to help them flow towards thriving rather than feeling like a failure as a mother or parent.

Different Ways of Working with Creativity

I have offered a client vignette before, showing how I use creative objects in my work with postpartum psychosis (Haynes, 2022b, 2023). This time,

I would like to explore the scope of a few other creative methods, suitable for both individual and group work, offering some suggestions of how these might be used. All sorts of mediums are possible: photographic diaries, painting, playdoh or drawing, creative writing, picture cards such as OH cards (decks of cards with pictures and words designed to stimulate creativity and communication) or postcards, sand trays, music, poetry, movement and dance are some examples. I encourage clinicians to use any method that comes as a flash of inspiration and whatever seems appropriate for the client to experience together. However, all methods must be explored, thought through and contracted for with the client before using them. This list is also not exhaustive and is designed to give a flavour of creative methods rather than a set of guidelines or rights and wrongs. Contract, explore, work with, play, experience, intuit. Whatever is needed in the moment.

Paralinguistics can offer precious unspoken information into pre-verbal experiences and trauma. For one client, noticing her body language helped to unlock previously 'unthought', yet bodily-held, childhood trauma from horrible, invasive surgery as a very young child. This trauma was hindering her pathway to parenthood. Her body would 'speak' of the trauma, with agitated movements, yet neither of us understood completely what her body was saying. Understanding came when she explored these movements with me and then with her parents, and they could fill some of the gap in knowledge about her childhood experience. This helped to unlock what had become tokophobia for this client and a real fear of sexual intimacy between herself and her partner.

Picture cards, such as OH cards, or a random selection of postcards, with different representations of faces, paintings or places chosen by the client can also be combined with words to increase insight and to help with communication between client and therapist. There are all manner of these cards on the market and the combinations are endless. They are suitable to be used in individual, couple or group therapy. Also, having an array of random magazines, scissors, large pads of blank paper and glue can also be a way to encourage clients to free associate through collage and pictures, rather than words. The collage can then be explored in the moment or in subsequent sessions. I have used collage work successfully when helping clients to unlock their feelings of loss and grief. Grief can often feel too deep to speak about, particularly if it is from the loss of a baby through stillbirth. Pictures can speak a thousand words when the client may feel unable to voice their loss.

Photographic diaries or a record of symbolic objects, which the client does on a weekly basis, can build into a representation of the client's affect, and may show movement and change, which might not have been recognised or seen without this visual record. Such a diary needs to be contracted for, thinking carefully about who can see or not, and who the diary is for (parent, infant, therapist). This contracting is important and ripe for exploration, as is the process of assembling the diary, particularly when drivers hinder the process.

Body movement can be particularly powerful in the perinatal, and more widely, in any form of client work. Movement can help with flow when a client feels particularly stuck or is experiencing PTSD symptoms or dissociation. I have even suggested clients put their feet into my sand tray and feel the sand with their toes as a way to help with dissociation and PTSD and possibly help them to link to positive childhood experiences like being on a beach. The act of movement and using the client's senses can be a form of break in the cycle of dissociative episodes. However, I would caution that some sensations can bring trauma sensations forward, so this needs to be thought through with the client, to ensure this does not happen.

I often suggest creative writing and drawing for clients to express their feelings and emotions, or to draw them using colour to depict them differently. Again, with clients who are experiencing high levels of grief and/or trauma, this can help them to show their emotions in a different way, and the use of their body through writing or drawing can mean their mind is more available for free association. I have also tried combining the two whereby the client has used particular colours of pen when writing to explore the depth of their feelings, offering a more nuanced version of their creative writing. Creative writing can work powerfully in groups with similar experiences, such as infertility. I was first introduced to the idea of creative writing as a tool in supervision by a TA psychotherapist called Anita Webster, through her Master's dissertation in 2020.

I use creative writing in supervision groups for clinicians working in perinatal psychotherapy. A supervisee will present their client and state what they want from supervision. As a group, we then spend a short time quietly free associating about the presented client, writing down whatever comes to mind. One by one, we then bring our thoughts and words back into the group and share them with the supervisee. The supervisee is then encouraged to explore these free associations and to co-create meaning about their client with the other group participants.

I also use free association in individual supervision. If the supervisee seems stuck or at a loss about a client, or if we both need to explore at a greater depth, I will ask them to free associate and give me the first object or colour they think of. It is important they do not spend too long thinking as this can hamper the process, and they can get caught in a trap of trying to please me by finding the 'perfect' object.

Free association often begins a process of slowly unearthing interesting and unspoken information about the client. For example, a supervisee shared an animal she thought of to represent the mother she was working with – a fox. We then explored the fox, what it represented about the client, what its character traits were, whether it was timid, aloof or aggressive. At this point, I would caveat not to lead the supervisee, as it is important for the free association to be theirs. However, it is possible to offer observations and thoughts, including any transferential feelings we notice, but not to force the process in any way. For the supervisee with the client whose object was a fox, this led to them uncovering their sense of the client as resourceful, and more competent and able than they had thought.

Another perinatal supervisee shared their stuckness around the case study client within their CTA dissertation. The supervisee felt bogged down, literally visualising themselves walking through treacle and quickly realised this was countertransference, that the client also felt bogged down and stuck in her low mood. This opened up an exploration of options the client might have to get out of the treacle bog: what she needed, how she could resource herself, what would make the treacle less sticky, so she was no longer stuck and could step out of it. "Walking through treacle" or being "stuck in the mud" are metaphors that often emerge with free association in the perinatal space. This parallels the process that parents can feel they are in – caught, mystified and at their wit's end.

I want to end with a few more caveats to creative work. When using movement and dance with a trauma client or with someone who may dissociate, it is helpful to negotiate what movements might be triggering and to contract carefully around what might be helpful if triggering occurs – whatever method is being used, ensuring that the therapist is not pushing the client, or trying to coerce or control them, which may enact something for the client. It is quite possible to miss the client by taking the process too fast into the non-verbal, which may provoke anxiety in the client. Finally, if the creative method does not seem to be working, then there may be a dissonance which may be more about the therapist's keenness to try the creative process, leaving the client feeling missed and unprepared.

Conclusion

By writing this chapter, I hope to inspire more TA practitioners to explore creative methods in whatever work they are in – psychotherapy, organisational work, training, supervision or teaching – as part of co-creative learning. I hope this chapter can spark thinking, contemplation and possibly the curiosity to give creativity a go. I hope you find your own explorations with it as useful as I have. I continue to probe and test how to use creative methods, processes and thinking, and in particular, to find meaning from my mistakes. Creativity continues to challenge and encourage me to never stop learning. I feel like I am still at the beginning of my creative journey, exploring and discovering its potential for perinatal psychotherapy and silence, and for me the future is exciting and rich with creative possibilities.

9

A JOINT ENDEAVOUR

Working with Couples

With contributions from Valeria Villa

How do we work effectively with couples in the perinatal sphere? What are the most common presentations in couples' therapy, and are there clues about why they are so common? How do we deal with a couple who seem at war in their relationship when a new baby is about to be born? What about helping a couple through cultural differences or disagreements about how their infant will be raised or their struggles with sexual intimacy after birth? There are many things to consider in couples work, and many themes and issues can arise. This chapter will explore some of the common themes and difficulties, will offer a few suggestions to open our minds to couples work and give some examples of this work.

I believe it would be useful for couples contemplating family life to come into therapy sooner rather than later, as a way of exploring their expectations, and to illuminate any differences in opinion, as a couple. At present, many parenting courses and ante-natal classes are offered and advertised. However, antenatal classes tend to focus only on the birth experience. Therapy can address much wider aspects, such as existential questions around parenting: Who do I want to be as a parent? Who influences me in my choice of parenting styles? What is most important to me and my partner when raising this child? Therapy in the antenatal period can make such a difference to couples, single mums, parents and fathers, and a therapeutic space can complement antenatal classes. It is so much easier to offer psychotherapeutic help to those embarking on their parenting journey before it has actually begun. Trying to patch up relationship difficulties, increase trust, and resolve money and childcare arguments once the infant has arrived is not an easy task, as there is already so much pressure trying to simply live as a family.

Many couples give so little thought and perhaps find it difficult to prioritise time to explore their parenting ideals, cultural norms or biases, and their own experiences of being parented. Becoming parents together is such a fundamental change in a couple's life. Yet, often, there seems to be an assumption that having children is simply a normal, natural step in a couple's journey, which does not need unpicking or unpacking. This may be true for some. However, for others, parenting can be tough even at the best of times, and exploring

DOI: 10.4324/9781003365822-9

the numerous factors involved can provide fertile areas of discussion, often unearthing differences between partners that are usefully aired before the arrival of their first child. Some examples of topics are: how the couple wants to co-parent; what they think about childcare; what type of childcare that might be (within the wider family or a nursery or childminding setting); who is expected to be the stay-at-home parent; what kind of education they want to give their children; and how they want to discipline their children.

In this chapter, I have attempted to be as gender-neutral as possible. In some parts, I have chosen to use the term mother or father to differentiate between the birthing or primary caregiver from the non-birthing, non-pregnant or non-primary caregiver or parent. This is because if I used the term parent, there might be confusion about which parent I was speaking about. Couples and families can be very diverse in type and style and can include many different types of parents. The focus of work is on the relationship between the couple to help them parent their infant as effectively as possible in the way that works best for them.

Couples: Bringing the Partner into the Sessions

When working one-to-one, usually with the mother, I always offer a session or two so the partner can attend as well. This is for several reasons: it helps the partner to feel included; they can ask me any questions they have; I can bust a few often-held myths; and I can clarify some aspects of the pregnancy, birth or post-birth process they did not want to or felt they should not ask their partner about.

Often, when the mother is struggling, the partner may feel unsure about what is happening and clueless about how to help. Her behaviour might seem dramatic, her anxiety may be through the roof, or perhaps the opposite is happening. She might remain silent about how she feels, cannot share anything with her partner, or even keeps saying nothing is wrong, even when it clearly is. For those used to an independent and efficient partner, a collapse in her efficiency, particularly post-birth, may seem out of character and concerning. She may seem obsessed with her new infant, unable to put them down, and her partner may find this baby-centric behaviour unnerving and might perceive it as excluding them, pushing them away. Being able to offer reassurance that it is not only normal but also natural for a mother to be preoccupied with her new infant can go a long way towards helping the couple begin to find some common ground and understand each other again.

Within these single couple sessions, topics that come up are often the partners' expectations of both the birth and post-birth life together and their thoughts on their inclusion during pregnancy, birth and within the infant's life. Sometimes, the expectations of both partners are at odds. An example of this is a partner who believed his wife should be able to 'get over' a termination for medical reasons (TFMR) and simply immediately try for another baby, discounting his wife's grief and the trauma of her experience. A man can never know what it feels like to be pregnant and then lose or choose to terminate the baby and how brutal and shaming this can feel. When a partner discounts in this way or tells the woman to "pull her socks up", this can be tricky to witness as a therapist, and confronting this behaviour also has its risks. I believe the risk needs to be taken. Yes, it may mean the couple choose not to come back. In this example, the husband began to understand that psychotherapy meant he also had to look at, explore and own his own behaviour. This can be too troubling, and hence, he stepped away and encouraged his wife into her own therapy without him. Perhaps he saw this as a way of bringing her into line with his position.

Other examples might be when a partner feels clueless about what is happening and does not recognise behaviours, or they perceive their partner (most usually the mother) as "acting out of character". In this respect, my role might be to help the partner understand more fully the normal and natural nature of these changes and help them to find compassion and empathy for the mother rather than judgement. The session is an opportunity to open up exploration about what is happening intrapsychically for the partner, which is clearly troubling them. This can help towards tolerance, both of the mother's experience and emotions and the rollercoaster of hormones she is experiencing, as well as of his own disturbance. Useful explorations can be around transgenerational influences on difference and otherness, and what is becoming agitated in our script messages (therapists and both partners).

It often comes as a huge surprise to both parents how much time and energy a newborn requires. Many couples don't seem to grasp that their infant will require 24/7 care and seem caught up in the mystification of the oft-portrayed happy, loving, nurturing family that lives the social media life of Facebook, Instagram and TikTok. The reality of an infant seeming to scream the house down day and night can be difficult to grasp, terrifying and hugely wearing, consuming all the energy the mother may have felt prior to pregnancy. Parenthood is transformative and not necessarily positive.

Psychoeducation can be helpful, particularly around birth trauma, psychosis, sexual dysfunction, sleep deprivation, physical damage in birth, intimacy post-birth and for numerous other topics from parenthood. Mostly, I find that partners want to understand what is happening and then want to know how they can help. Some women are so ashamed of how they feel they remain silent and secretive and do not share any of their experience with their partner or close family members, so it can come as a bit of a shock when there is a realisation of just how unwell she might be.

It is important to state that this single session does need to be with both parents together, as a couple, but doesn't necessarily need to be more than one session and two at the most. This is enough time to help the couple come together and talk about their concerns. It also gives them an opportunity to be more open and honest with each other, which goes a long way towards opening communication channels, gaining understanding and unlocking a level of compassion and empathy so that they might begin to offer each other some emotional and psychological relief.

However, it is vital to contract with your primary client beforehand, drawing out any of the details that can be shared or need to be withheld so boundaries can be kept and the therapist does not inadvertently speak about something the client does not want to share. I also like to ask if there are any fears about having the partner in the session, what the expectations are about my role, and if there are any particular things that I need to say or highlight. This contracting is so important. It allows the session to be as transparent and effective as possible.

Reticence

Some women can be hesitant or even reticent about inviting their partner into a session with them. Concerns might be whether it will change our relationship (therapist and client), whether the partner will listen, or perhaps even a fear that the partner will be defensive and dismissive towards me. Whatever the reason, it is important to dig into and explore the reticence. In some cases, it has transpired that my client is concerned that their portrayal of their partner might have been 'wrong', or that their partner will manipulate me. Many clients I see, particularly those whom I begin to sense a level of control or manipulation from their partners, are concerned that I won't be 'strong enough' to see through the charm and manipulation. In these instances, it can be beneficial to explore what is behind the reticence and whether this is hiding some deeper difficulties in the relationship.

What if the reticence is mine? There have been some occasions when it was not appropriate to include the partner. For example, there may be a concern that the partner is quite controlling, and likely to talk at me during the session, or would take over or shut down and marginalise the mother's voice. If this is the case, inviting him into the session may not help the situation and may exacerbate his need for control. He may also feel like he is being invited in to be told how to behave or act by me (another woman), even if that is not my intention at all.

Regardless of whose reticence it is, mine, my client's or their partner's, it is helpful to really dig down into unconscious processes and explore what is really going on. Supervision, particularly with a group of peers, can be really helpful in these instances, as there is often a difference or multitude of opinions that may tease out some hidden messages or behaviours.

My client, Hannah, was not at all sure about her partner joining us, and I was curious about this. Hannah originally came after the birth of her first child, Mabel, because she was struggling with perfectionism. She was now pregnant with her second child, another girl, and I suggested inviting her husband, Paul, into a session before the birth. Yet, Hannah was not at all keen.

I wondered about her reticence and felt this needed further exploration. I was unclear whether she was concerned about Paul being in the session with us or whether she felt more in control, perhaps, without him there. What began as her defensiveness about him – "he is too busy", "he won't commit himself to a time", "he doesn't want to be involved" – in reality was her fear of loss of control, and also shame about the return of her perfectionism, which Hannah could not bear to admit to herself. Her fear was that Paul would have spoken about her perfectionism and then I would have known.

What I knew of Hannah, in our work together, was that she felt the need to be in control, and this led her to putting her child first in everything, leaving Hannah at the bottom of the pile. This was now occurring to such an extent that Hannah finally admitted to spending hours late at night, doing what she called "doom-scrolling" on social media, looking for clothes for Mabel and checking to ensure that her daughter was the best in comparison to her friends' children.

What I also realised was that Hannah was excluding Paul from the life she and Mabel had together, although when I drew this to her attention, she denied it. When I challenged her and asked why she was blocking Paul from a session together, she was able to finally admit her fear that if he came to the session, he might actually tell me how much time Hannah was spending on what Paul called her "obsession". Unpacking this reticence offered the chance for Hannah and I to focus our attention back onto her perfectionism, and what this was hiding – her fear of having a second child, that she could not possibly "love as much" as her first, but also her fear about having to divide herself between two children.

A Joint Endeavour?

Questions that might come up in these joint sessions with the partner may be about things such as feeding – will the mother be breastfeeding totally, or might she consider expressing some milk so her partner can be included in a feed or two each day? Would she want her partner to be present at night-time feeds? Is this practical? What other areas could they help with? Does the partner feel comfortable doing nappy changes and looking after the baby if she is absent? How does she feel about leaving them with the baby? Conversely, how do they feel about being left alone with the baby? All of these questions might appear insignificant, yet for the mother and partner, there may be differing levels of fear and concern.

I am surprised how many partners feel they cannot ask questions due to not wanting to bother the mother or perhaps are concerned that their fears or worries might not be taken seriously, or that this will diminish them in some way in the mother's eyes. Some partners remain silent, feeling excluded or even isolated from the birth process. This silence is not helpful for a couple and can be a clue that the couple might benefit from couples' therapy to help them connect and communicate more fruitfully post-birth.

What is all too apparent is that often the partner does not realise they have much of a role to play in those first few weeks and months of life with a newborn, believing that the mother is the one who needs to or should be the main carer. Helping partners understand their importance can help them feel included and part of the birth process, rather than being excluded and feeling like a nuisance or spare part. For instance, their role may be as an advocate for their partner during birth, so including them in some sessions before the birth can help to highlight what they can advocate for. It allows discussion about how they might speak up, for example, if they are concerned about the treatment their partner is receiving or if they are concerned their partner is not receiving what she needs. This is particularly important for mothers from Black, Asian or minority ethnic groups, due to how often they are not heard, or are dismissed or discounted during pregnancy, birth and post-birth. In these instances, having a partner who can advocate vocally for better care can be the difference between life and death. A useful place to start for male partners is with a very well-researched and readable book by Anna Machin called *The Life of Dad – the Making of the Modern Father.*

Couples Work

Couples quite often come into therapy together before a baby arrives, perhaps due to relationship or infertility issues such as those couples embarking on different types of ART, such as IVF. Regardless of when or why they come, one of the biggest themes in couples work is discounting. This discounting can occur for many reasons and might be due to the couple not quite grasping the gap between their fantasy of family life and the reality once the baby is born, a common theme with new parents. It might be due to the trauma of miscarriage or stillbirth, and discounting can occur when coupled with a Hurry Up in the non-pregnant partner. Another theme that seems to indicate a level of discounting is around the role of the mother-in-law, which may become problematic, particularly around the arrival of the baby. Also, one or both partners may be discounting vulnerability in one or even both of them, and this discounting may deepen when the enormity of the responsibility begins to become a reality for the couple. Discounting is such a useful theory with application in both perinatal and couples work and is easily grasped by couples. Other useful TA theories are the drama triangle (Karpman, 1968) coupled with the winner's triangle (Choy, 1990), interlocking scripts (Holtby, 1979; Parkin, 2014), the shame loop (Little, 1999) and ego state theory.

Discounting

Let's explore a few of the most common time periods when discounting seems most likely to occur. With a heteronormative couple, tensions might arise around the differences in the masculine and feminine roles within the relationship, and this can happen in cross-cultural relationships. For example, when the woman gives birth, some men can feel a level of envy towards the new power the woman appears to have. With single-sex and gender-neutral couples, a similar process can occur when the birth parent and infant gain a huge amount of attention during the birth process. The focus of attention from family and friends, midwives and medical staff is on their care, and sometimes the non-birthing partner can feel left out or sidelined.

The responsibility towards their partner and new child can bring a great deal of fear and trepidation for partners. In my experience, partners, and in particular men, can find it difficult to express how they feel, particularly if their feelings are overwhelming and scary. They might not have contemplated how enormous this responsibility would feel, and this can bring concerns about their new role. When the non-birthing partner is not secure in their own sense of self, this newfound weight of responsibility has the potential to impact them.

Fears that come up for both parents in couples therapy are often around the health of the baby, such as what if the baby is born disabled (Erikssen, Westman & Hamberg, 2005), is stillborn or dies in childbirth (Etheridge & Slade, 2017; Shibli-Kometiani & Brown, 2013. Other fears can be concerns for the mother, such as whether something might happen to her, and will she cope with the pain of childbirth (Greer, Lazenbatt & Dunne, 2014). Some men doubt their own capacity and are fearful of fainting or panicking during childbirth (Somers-Smith, 1999 or fear their inability to support their partner during labour (Greer et al., 2014). All of these instances can increase both partners' fears about childbirth, particularly with a first child or if there has been prior birth trauma.

When partners find talking about their fears of childbirth and parenting difficult to express, couples therapy can give them space to voice these fears so that the mother can hear about them. Some men state that societal expectations are such that it is up to them to remain strong and be the protector (Moran et al., 2021). It is common for men to have a Be Strong driver. When both partners have a fear of childbirth, exploring and working out how they can support each other can be really fruitful prior to birth. Around 13% of men have a fear of childbirth (Erikssen, Salander & Hamberg, 2007; Hildingsson et al., 2014), bringing with it severe anxiety, feelings of helplessness, and shame. For women between 10 and 20% will have a fear of childbirth that needs exploration and investigation (Rublein & Muschalla, 2022).

Fear of an inability to breastfeed is another common difficulty and may come to light in couples, as well as individual therapy. For women desperate to breastfeed, finding out that this may not be possible post-birth can be experienced as an existential trauma (Palmér, 2019). When this happens, the woman needs the partner to be supportive of her, not to try and make it ok, by discounting the impact on her. Some women are fearful of breastfeeding and do not want to try it. Getting help with establishing breastfeeding is crucial in the earliest few days and weeks, and partners can support this, particularly if this is an area of discussion prior to the birth.

Other difficulties of discounting occur due to lack of knowledge. For example, when a woman experiences postpartum psychosis, her partner may be extremely shocked that this has occurred and may find it difficult to process. Psychosis comes with so much stigma and myth that some men become terrified of their partner, normally due to a lack of useful information from medical staff about what is actually happening and how to offer appropriate help. Discounting the severity of the psychosis, and in particular, discounting the time it may take to come through this traumatic experience, is also common. The couple's work might initially be about helping the father find compassion and empathy after the psychosis is over and to help him be realistic about the pathway ahead. There can be a tendency to believe that once mother and baby leave the care of the inpatient psychiatric mother and baby unit, the worst is over, but this is not at all true. Both parents may need help to process what has happened. Couples can fall apart after such an experience due to the trauma involved. Yet helping the couple to communicate about the trauma can be a healing process and help both to feel more connected, reminding them that they both experienced this.

This is similar to experiences of birth trauma. It is easy to forget that the partner may have experienced vicarious trauma from watching the birth, seeing and hearing it happening in real-time. Getting the couple to talk about their experience in therapy and offering space for the partner to admit the terror they felt can be an intimate experience. For example, a partner experienced their newborn infant struggling to breathe and thought the infant would die, but at the same time, the mother was also extremely sick, and their genuine fear was that they would lose both, but felt helpless to intervene in any way. Many partners find it almost impossible to talk about these types of experiences and to admit their terror, and horror, holding onto these secrets, which can eat away at them and impact their sense of self.

There are more discounting examples in a later section of this chapter on cross-cultural difficulties.

Lack of Trust

What happens when one parent doesn't trust the other? One thing that can occur is that the parent with trust issues can become a barrier between the child and the other parent. Sadly, divorce shows this quite literally, as many parents face being restricted from their child or children due to mistrust from the other parent, and as a form of punishment for the end of the relationship.

In couples' therapy, this mistrust needs to be challenged so that there is space to bring to the fore what is real and what is fantasy. Asking what is being activated in the withholding parent can bring to light why they feel so unsafe and can highlight some of the behaviours that may be creating these feelings of a lack of safety. Sometimes a parent is avoidant, or even gives up in the face of criticism and withdraws from helping to care for their infant. One parent might seem to be unaware of basic infant safety, which might transpire to be a cultural difference. For example, an Italian father with quite a laissez-faire attitude towards safety who did not consider the efficacy of the car seat important, with an attitude that children were much more robust than we give them credit for and would survive okay. Unfortunately, his wife, who was from Sweden, known for its safety-conscious nature, had a very different idea of what was okay and reported feeling a deep mistrust of his care towards their infant.

Perhaps there is a grain of truth behind whatever mistrust is there. Nevertheless, parenting is a joint role, and it is important to explore where the mistrust stems from. Exploring whether it may be part of a person's script or from the person's own experience of being parented can help to reduce the mistrust and prevent it from becoming a barrier to connection.

Another area ripe for mistrust is baby-led weaning or food in general. Perhaps the food is a metaphor for something else within the couple's relationship, and their connection needs to become the actual focus of the work. Food can bring up all manner of control issues. For example, Leah was obsessed about being in control of her daughter's food, because she was terrified that the child would become "fat". Leah would not allow anyone to feed her, and took all her own homemade food to nursery, to social events they went to as a family, and even to a family event. Leah had a fear that her daughter would eat "the wrong thing". This was a serious problem for her and her partner, Andy. Once they were able to have space to talk about what was going on, Leah's fear of her daughter's weight transpired as her own fear of being overweight, and no longer attractive to Andy. Once Andy reassured Leah about how he perceived her, this allowed them to stop fighting over food, and allowed them more space to focus on their daughter rather than continuing the fight.

As a brief aside, if there are concerns that a couple may be arguing to the detriment of their children, or that the children are at risk from violence, there may well be safeguarding issues that would need to be aired, both in supervision and with the couple. It is also useful to ensure that there is knowledge of the rules regarding physical punishment of children in the country in which the couple live (both for the therapist and the couple).

Barry and David came into therapy as parents of two small children. They wanted to try and remain together, despite struggling due to David's perception of Barry's "bad behaviour". David didn't trust Barry with their children and found it difficult to leave them alone with him. Barry was angry and quite confused as he didn't really understand why he was not to be trusted and felt that David was becoming a barrier between Barry and the boys.

What transpired was that both came from very different backgrounds and grew up experiencing completely different styles of parenting. What David perceived as untrustworthy behaviour might be considered normal in other families. David admitted that his parents were overly protective and found it difficult to let him go when he was growing up. In contrast, Barry's parents wanted him to explore and "stand on his own two feet", and he was encouraged to be self-sufficient from an early age.

Barry wanted to try and inspire a similar level of responsibility and autonomy in his own children, yet David found this behaviour deeply unsettling and worrying. He didn't understand why any parent would want to encourage their child to be independent. He was used to parenting that sounded quite symbiotic and dependent. Therapy involved exploring many different types of parenting, what each might mean for the child and what both Barry and David wanted for their boys. Inevitably, they wanted the same things: for the boys to be happy and secure. Once they began to see how similar their hopes were, the mistrust in David began to diminish and he found ways of beginning to trust Barry's judgement and parenting skills and could accept it was ok for these to be different.

Gender Equality and Co-Parenting

Couples may come to therapy with co-parenting issues, which may come to light, particularly after the birth of a baby. These difficulties may stem from tensions around gender equality, and differing opinions on parenting roles. In this case, it may be worth exploring historical messages about gender and childcare, which may linger in the background both consciously and unconsciously. These historical messages can bring patterns of behaviour that may seem stereotypical and outdated yet still exist.

According to the World Bank, in 2022, more than 50% of women now work in the labour force as opposed to 80% of men. In the US, in 2022, both parents were employed in 48.9% of married-couple families (World Bank 2022b; Bureau of Labor Statistics, 2023). In the UK, in 2021, 57.7% of families with one child had both parents working full-time and 75.7% of mothers with dependent children were working (ONS, 2022a). In the EU in 2021, 72% of women aged between 25 and 54 with children were working. Again, in the EU in 2021, 57.9% of households with children who were economically dependent had both parents working (European Commission, 2022).

In Asia and the Pacific, there is a very mixed pattern of women entering and leaving the labour force before, during and after childbirth. In Japan and Korea, for example, and less so in Australia and New Zealand, female employment rates fall between 30 and 39 years of age and then rebound from around 45 years of age, which may indicate that in these countries, women might leave the labour force when they have children and then rejoin it afterwards. In China and Thailand, there is little change between 30 and 39 years of age and yet in others, like Singapore, women seem to leave the labour market completely from 30 to 34 (OECD, 2021).

Why is this relevant? It is clear that many more women worldwide are now working full-time or are employed in some way. Yet some attitudes and behaviours have not caught up. Women also have lower incomes from work and are more often expected to work for free. And it is well known that, in general, women do not have the same opportunities in their careers as men. However, this is not an excuse for any expectation that women should be the main carers of children. This seems to remain unspoken or is swept under the carpet by many couples and in many cultures. Yet, with so many parents now working, these are conversations couples need to have, preferably prior to the arrival of children. This is especially important because equality within a partnership is seen as a requirement for contemporary relationships to be successful (Knudson-Martin & Mahoney, 2009).

It is known that the emotional health of children is higher when both parents prioritise family above and beyond work, due to the parent's physical and emotional availability to the child (Friedman, 2018). Parenting is a two-person job, and thus, if there are two parents available, this should not be forgotten. One useful part of therapy can be highlighting the joint responsibilities in parenting and challenging both partners' ideas on the burden of care within their relationship. For some couples and in some cultures, it is entirely natural and normal that the woman should be the main caregiver to the children. However, within the industrialized world, there is a definite move towards greater gender equality (Sullivan 2006). Being creative, and getting the couple to literally place markers on a table in front of them, each describing a task that needs to be done in the house, for the children and within the family, then discussing these markers regarding capability, playing to each partner's strengths in the relationship, can begin to help the couple physically see the inequitable division of those responsibilities. It is also a little harder for one partner to deny what is occurring when it is literally in front of them.

The move towards gender equality within romantic relationships seems to have brought with it a fragility to some relationships (Knudson-Martin & Mahoney, 2009), with both partners often having quite high standards of the other. This can cause difficulties, particularly if there is an intolerance to some types of behaviours. According to research by Coontz (2005), many women said they are no longer willing to tolerate inequality and will not shoulder the burden of chores and caregiving, and men said they are no longer willing to tolerate weakness or subservience in their female partners. This can cause stuckness and tension between partners and a sense of ongoing inequalities of power. It is important to confront and challenge both the stuckness and the power dynamics, as some of this may come from historic or cultural gender disparities, which are sat firmly in the background. Also, shedding light on one partner exercising power over the other is useful as this type of behaviour is not helpful and may cause relationship breakdown (Greenberg & Goldman, 2008), which is not a good environment in which to raise a small infant.

The arrival of a newborn infant can also be a time when dysfunctional relationship norms come to light, including all those tricky behaviours that both partners knew about the other, but perhaps had swept under the carpet before departing on the parenting journey. Any form of unwillingness in one or both partners to look at these issues and resolve them can begin a spiral into future relationship breakdown. It is difficult to air these things, yet the relationship is normally much stronger once this can happen.

Driver Behaviour

As said earlier, it is quite common for a man to have a Be Strong driver. This is not necessarily a problem and can be helpful if the mother needs an advocate or someone to take charge if she is not well or is struggling with bonding. For parents with twins, this can be such an overwhelming time, that one partner with a Be Strong driver is very useful. However, if the other then has a Be Perfect driver and they are both people pleasers, the people pleasing can really get in the way of the relationship. This can cause problems between the couple as there is often a fear of confronting what is really happening in case the other gets hurt, leading to resentment and a possible lack of trust. This niceness in both can result in the couple going around in circles and as a therapist, this can be difficult to experience. It is also a significant barrier to intimacy in the couple and may be seriously hampering the couple's sex life.

A Be Strong driver can so often be linked with a Try Hard driver, and the two can be an absolute killer for a mother, particularly if there is also a bit of perfectionism lurking in the background. So many times I have experienced mothers who feel they have to do everything; who cannot rest, and who seem to hold the burden of the world on their shoulders. These mothers try so hard to be on it all the time with their families. They are normally extremely efficient and seem to be able to remember everything their child needs. On the flip side, they can seem engulfing; they often do not allow their child to fail, and they may spend hours at night, to the detriment of their sleep, organising and preparing for the next days and weeks, or even completing doing their child's homework. The other parent can become resentful of the lack of intimacy (there is always something that needs to be done that gets in the way, not to mention the tiredness and lack of sleep) and the time spent on what may be considered trivial, unimportant tasks.

A Be Perfect driver in the female is really common. Throughout this book, I have spoken about perfectionism and how hampering this can be in the maternal journey. Unfortunately, there is so much portrayal of what some perceive as the perfect family in social media, television and film productions and in magazines and journal articles, that expectations of life post-birth can become skewed. This desire to show the world what a perfect life mother and baby are having together can be unreal and also unhealthy. It may help to make the mother feel like she is in control of something in her and her infant's life, but the reality is often far from the truth. Perfectionism in a mother needs to be confronted as it is closed-loop behaviour. Child-rearing is messy, untidy, sometimes boring and often chaotic and all parents make mistakes. It can also have wonderful moments, and most parents would not change it for the world. Making mistakes is important as a parent, particularly if the parent is able to admit their mistakes and learn from them, doing it differently next time. This is very helpful for a child to see modelled. The continual need to portray how glorious and perfect family life is sets everyone in the family up to fail, and that failure is often hugely painful.

Being the partner of someone with a Be Perfect driver can be infuriating and worrying. I will come to money in a moment, but there can be a real fear that perfectionism takes over everything else, to the detriment of the connection between the couple, and also the connection between mother and child. No child, once they begin to grow up, wants to be the Facebook pin-up, having their photo taken left, right and centre and then plastered all over group chats or social media to be used to fulfil the mother's needs. The partner may also be concerned about this behaviour and want to voice their concern but not feel able to. They might be concerned that later on in life, the child will really resent their life being subject to social scrutiny. Also, once the photos are on social media it is almost impossible to remove them, regardless of what the child wants.

With regard to money, if one partner does not approve of spending money, and the other is a perfectionist, this can cause huge problems and breakdowns in trust. The perfectionist partner may insist that some parenting paraphernalia is essential to their infant's life, yet the other may perceive it as a ridiculous frippery or absolutely unnecessary, so bust-ups can occur, and trust begins to fade away.

Hurry Up, as I mentioned earlier, will rear its head when one partner believes the other needs to "get on with", "get over" or "get through" whatever it is they have experienced. It also comes up with couples desperate to become pregnant, but who are struggling with fertility issues. For these couples, it is almost as if they have an hourglass in the background, with the sand inexorably slipping away. Every month, when they have not conceived the time gets less, and the sand seems to ebb away even faster. Or perhaps, just one partner has this sense, and the other partner is the opposite and has a need to pause for the moment. This can be a difficult situation to navigate for a couple and may risk fracturing the relationship or causing resentment.

Hurry Up can manifest itself towards the child too, when the parent walks at a pace that the child has to jog to keep up with, or with a competitive parent who expects the child to be doing things as early as possible. This can seem quite performative, as if the parent is doing parenting for the sake of it rather than actually allowing the child to be.

Just a brief word on injunctions. Obviously, many injunctions are active in couples work. In particular, within a couple, Don't Be You in one parent can be reinforced by the other. Equally, it is also possible that this injunction is internalised from the person's history, through transgenerational scripting, or even internalised from society.

Value: Money

How do the couple value each other, and where do they allocate household resources? Who gives up work? Do they put their infant into childcare? How do they come to an agreement about this, and does one partner hold more power than the other? If they are both working, who takes time off when a child is inevitably sick and cannot go to childcare or school? This is such a big deal for couples and can bring up so many arguments.

The non-birthing partner may be really concerned about having to provide for the family and fearful that they may not be able to. For those who didn't have good role models with money growing up, this fear can feel overwhelming, and they may feel like they are bound to repeat the same mistakes. How does this get addressed in the couple, and what has becoming a family thrown up around money and value?

If one person wants to save money, and the other is merrily spending it, this can be a massive difficulty, as noted before. What about if they need help from a cleaner or a babysitter, for example? Who pays? Who gets the benefit? Who is in charge of them and organises when they come to help out? What if a couple chooses to place their infant in the care of a nursery? It may seem cheaper and a way to economise (although in some countries, like the UK, for example, nurseries are prohibitively expensive) rather than choosing to have a nanny, but what about the long-term benefits for the infant and the family as a whole? For example, neither parent would need to take time off work if the infant is ill when there is a nanny. Yet the infant would not be able to attend nursery.

If one parent is staying at home to look after the children, how are they valued, and how do they get paid for their role? In the US, research by Salary.com (2019) tracking all the tasks a mother does in her day, using real-time costs of that work, put the median value of a stay-at-home mother at $178,201 per annum. Even if this is overstated, it still helps couples to begin to think about the value of the stay-at-home parent. Money is such an emotive topic for so many couples and can be at the heart of perinatal couples' therapy.

What about money and value when the couple is experiencing fertility difficulties and needs to spend money on fertility treatment? Another cause for resentment may be the amount of time and money that is being invested, and if the couple are struggling to afford the treatment, navigating the debt and finding ways to cope with it, once the child is born, can cause difficulties, too. This can cause a rift between the couple, especially if one partner is 'at fault' for being infertile. There may be some expectation for the 'faulty' partner to somehow 'pay' or even 'repay' the fertile partner.

Cross-Cultural Difficulties

I have spoken about some cross-cultural difficulties in this chapter. However, it warrants a section as a way to pause and explore some of the difficulties that can arise with parents from different cultures. Things to explore prior to the child being born might be:

Language: Which language will we speak to our child? Will this be the same language or different to the language we speak to each other? What if we speak for example, Italian at home, but we live in the UK, and the two sets of grandparents speak different languages too? How do we navigate language together? Whose language is the most important?

Religion: Again, whose religion is most important, whose do we discount? How do we negotiate religious holidays that are important in one culture but not in another (Christmas, Easter, etc.).

Culture: What culture do we highlight? What about nursery rhymes and fairy tales from the two different cultures? Which books will we read to our children?

Practices: How do these get negotiated, for example, circumcision?

This list is not exhaustive. There are so many issues that can appear, many of which have never been a problem prior to parenthood. Couples who are from different cultures may have worked really well until the point at which they fall pregnant. This can be when a crucial bond of loyalty to one's culture can suddenly materialise, even when it had not existed prior. Having a child is such an emotional time, and this sense of 'home' or even 'homeland' can become so important for both partners, bringing the need to show the child where they come from, sharing their language, their religion and their ancestry, and also as part of belonging.

It is also a time when existential fear can set in, in all sorts of ways. For example, a mother who stated that she had felt "colour-blind" to her partner's skin colour, and said she had suddenly developed an awareness of the "shade" her baby might be once it was born, and did not know how to address this, or speak of her fear to him. Or a mother married to a Chinese partner who gave birth to a girl, when he desperately wanted a boy. This led the mother to feel overly protective of their daughter and quite resentful of her husband, not allowing him time with the child in case he dismissed her.

Cross-cultural difficulties can cause all manner of problems. Again, having the opportunity to explore some of the issues the couple have come across (and have not even contemplated) can be really helpful in the contemplation stage, so that these do not materialise in the way they might later on.

The Mother-in-Law

The role of the respective mothers-in-law can also be a tension between couples, and particularly for those who come from different cultural experiences. One husband discounted the difficulty his mother presented to his wife. The husband had never really grown up properly and needed to please his mother and would find himself agreeing to her controlling demands. She lived in another country, so this did not pose too many difficulties unless she came to visit. However, just before their first baby's due date, the mother-in-law began to insist she was flying over so she could help out once the baby arrived. The mother-in-law never asked her daughter-in-law if help was wanted or needed. Instead, this was a cultural expectation held by the mother-in-law, as it was customary in her culture for a daughter-in-law to be living with the husband's parents. The mother-in-law could not understand why her coming was a problem, instead believing the daughter-in-law should be appreciative and humble towards her. However, she and the wife had never got on, and the wife found her behaviours towards her son demanding and frankly irritating. This became the topic of a great deal of upset in the couple, and their arguments became more heated the closer the due date got.

In therapy, the tension he felt between pleasing his mother and his wife was challenged, leading to an exploration of how his relationship with his mother had been when he was a boy (a protector of her from his violent and abusive father). He had not recognised that he was choosing his mother over his wife and child and was clueless about his wife's feelings, finding her arguments against his mother quite ridiculous and rude.

However, he began to recognise that by trying to please his mother, he was undermining the intimacy and connection with his wife and that she felt shunned and unimportant, leading her to feel unsafe and insecure in the marriage and to think about separation prior to the birth of their baby. He was shocked that she wanted to separate and began to see the depth of his wife's despair and how close he was to losing both his wife and unborn infant because he was unable to confront his symbiotic relationship with his mother.

Luckily, the husband was willing to work hard in couples' therapy, was able to own his part in the marital breakdown and realised how difficult it was for his wife to be second best to his mother. This helped him to see he needed to make a choice – wife and baby or mother.

Conclusion

Couples work can be fruitful in whatever stage of parenting. During contemplation it is a time when many difficulties can be brought out from under the carpet and tensions can be explored and resolved. Cultural difficulties and differences in opinion can also be highlighted and explored.

Whether it is through a single, psychoeducational session close to the baby's due date, or whether the couple come from the start or even before contemplating having a family, this type of therapy can be hugely helpful in strengthening the bond and support between the couple.

10

FREEDOM FROM ISOLATION
Working with Groups

With contributions from Valeria Villa and Sarah Crowley

How can we work with perinatal groups, and is the work similar or different to other TA group work? What ethical implications exist about working with such groups that may materialise and need consideration? Group work is such a fundamental part of TA, and it is possible to offer groups for all sorts of topics in perinatal work. I want to explore the value of group work within this area, as some types of groups don't seem to work. Through many failures, I have discovered that groups for perinatal low mood and/or anxiety are not well attended. Participants already have so much shame and fear that many won't consider any form of group work at all, and the mere thought of joining may bring feelings of panic. However, as with any form of group experience, it can help enormously with the isolation that so many parents and, particularly, mothers feel. Thought and care go a long way towards finding a suitable pathway into a group space. For mothers who might struggle with joining, working on a one-to-one basis first, addressing their maternal anxiety, shame and low self-esteem can be a beneficial first step into them joining a group process.

Groups can be for many different and specific parenting difficulties. They can also be useful in organisations (such as groups around miscarriage, advocacy, groups focused on changing the corporate attitude towards parenting, lobby groups for breastfeeding spaces, miscarriage and even menopause) and within educational settings too. Examples of successful groups are: the experience of going through IVF (groups for men, for women, and for single-sex couples); a fathers' and partners' group; a group for trainee therapists who were also parents; a fertility group aimed at older women; the experience of miscarriage and childlessness and how this might impact work and the support needed from the organisation; parenting children with friends or acquaintances rather than intimate partners; and although not in the perinatal sphere, coping with the menopause in a working environment. Numerous types of groups are possible due to the considerable breadth and depth of perinatal work.

It sounds self-evident, yet perinatal group work is not necessarily the same as standard group therapy. There are many elements of the group to be thought through before it commences. Flexibility is an important aspect to

DOI: 10.4324/9781003365822-10

both speak of and contract for. Defining the limits to flexibility and permeability are key elements when working in the perinatal field. This is because each member of the group is never just one person. For example, if it is a mother's group, there will be at least one child and often a partner who may impact the group and the mother's flexibility to attend. This is true of baby loss groups, too, because the lost infant needs to be accounted for and must not be discounted by and within the group.

Flexibility becomes a crucial issue with ante-natal groups, because when pregnant there are so many different appointments to attend. There are also deadlines for all sorts of things that can get in the way of group attendance. Post-birth, the child may be in the group space, or there may be childcare issues, school pickup deadlines, or child sickness to deal with. Mothers hold so much in their minds – pre-birth life, post-birth life, child, children, partner, relationships. All of these elements have schedules, so finding a suitable day and time can be tricky. It may also mean the group has many layers of complexity. The contracting stage will be between each of the attendees and the therapist and also between group members.

Valeria Villa, who is highly experienced in this type of work, highlights this aspect of working with groups of mothers and parents, and expresses the importance of continually returning to these aspects of flexibility and permeability in the contract. She recognises this as a parallel process to the parenting journey and draws attention to how these aspects may make the group feel lacking in a solid foundation and can be quite challenging. She told me she has needed to find the capacity to state a healthy "no" at times. For her, a guiding principle in this exploration is "who is this for?" Valeria says she continually wonders who is being accommodated, when she agrees to flexibility or when the group agrees. This is worth considering in supervision as a way of uncovering unconscious processes and perhaps script behaviour in the therapist.

Contracting is key in all manner of groups. In fertility groups, for instance, what might need to be contracted for, as opposed to infertility groups? Are there ethical implications for working in a group instead of individually with a client and how might this impact the contracting process? How might these implications be resolved? When offering a group for new mums, is it okay for them to bring their infants, too? How might this work, and how might the group dynamic change? Is online okay, or is face-to-face better when working with mothers and their infants? Is it a good idea to cap the group number? Due to the shame and stigma, should these be closed groups only, to keep any shame or stigma within the group and to help with the containment and boundaries?

As stated earlier, the therapist needs to think carefully about the group's purpose and who it is for, which needs to be clear at the outset, as does the aim. Things to think about are: is this a therapy group, is it a group with a shared experience (including the therapist's) in which the expectation is that all members share, or is it an emotional support group? Each of these is a very different style of group, with different aims.

As with any group, care needs to be taken around one person taking over or becoming the spokesperson, seeming to take up valuable space and time, leaving others silenced. If the outspoken group member is not contained, other group members may feel abandoned in their process by the therapist. For inexperienced group therapists, this can happen. For perinatal women, this abandonment may be a re-enactment of the silencing they have experienced in other spaces. Finding ways to contain this person without shaming them can be difficult. A word of warning: this can also happen when two therapists co-lead a group. One of the therapists can take over, leaving the other silent, which may, of course, be a re-enactment of a parenting experience around power and control.

Discounting can play a considerable part in group work, too. Discussions can surface and may be discounted through humour, among other things. Body shape comes to mind, as many women still have to buy clothes in much larger sizes, many months post-birth and can have difficulty in finding clothes to wear. These comments can be perceived as pragmatic about the post-birth reality. However, if there is humour, what is it covering? Many women become hugely anxious about their weight both pre and post-birth. Confronting this group discounting is very important.

Therapeutic holding and witnessing can also be essential aspects of perinatal groups. This applies, in particular, to those group members who have no real chance of change in their experience – for example, members of an infertility group or a perinatal loss and bereavement group. These elements, holding and witnessing, can be helpful to group members who may be desperate to feel less isolated in their loss and grief and to know they are not the only one. What almost certainly will change is the group members' ability to tolerate their experience, even if there is no hope of it changing as such.

Dilemmas can arise in all sorts of groups. For example, in a fertility group, over time group members became pregnant, leaving one who was not. This woman was left feeling shame and a sense of brokenness for being the only one not pregnant. What then? How might the therapist approach this? The group may want to move on, yet all of them will recognise the agony of infertility for this one woman, knowing full well that they are part of a 'club' that she so desperately wants to join, yet cannot. Perinatal work can be overwhelming for the therapist and for the group members, too, and there are so many dilemmas that can emerge. In group work, the possibility of these dilemmas surfacing rises exponentially.

As an example, what about a pregnancy support group for those who might want to explore their experiences with others who are also pregnant? The group members will likely gain a level of togetherness in their experience and may feel less alone and isolated. However, it is surprising how quickly a subtle undercurrent of competition can enter the group space. Much like there is often competition between mothers around milestones their child has met, this can be true of a group of pregnant women. Particularly when sharing stories of their difficulties in conceiving. Sometimes, it can be challenging to hold the group, not letting the topic slip into a frenzy of over-sharing and re-traumatisation.

What if the therapist becomes pregnant? Should the therapist pause her role in the group? Is that ethical? Would it be ethical to continue through her pregnancy? Do some group members have an expectation of the therapist sharing her experiences, or might it be a shock for them to realise that she, too, is pregnant? What might change in the group dynamics? Might the participants feel concerned, or might they feel this was appropriate and that when the therapist speaks, she comes from a place of experience?

What if the therapist is a mother or father themselves? What if they do not have adequate space for their own support? They are also at risk of burnout, as they may be trying to help the helpers, with groups for therapists who are also parents, which may become an impossible task for themselves. Burnout is an area I discuss in Chapter 12. Supervision is a critical part of the group work experience for therapists. Hopefully, the supervisor has experience of this type of work, although that is not a prerequisite.

A Perinatal Fertility Group

Sarah Crowley works with groups of women considering motherhood and also groups for assisted fertility treatments. She highlights how many online forums and websites there are, with women trading fertility stories, usually under pseudonyms, to offer solace and advice, and seek support as they move through what can be a challenging process. Many of these women also need to show up for work and family life and to try to continue friendships, social lives and commitments as well as going through the process of trying to become pregnant. This journey can be particularly arduous and may bring tension around family and friends. Assisted fertility, in particular, is so often cloaked in secrecy and shame because it is not seen as normal. Whilst online forums exist to try to help, they are not necessarily the only answer.

Sarah advocates groups to provide a sense of identification with others who are in similar circumstances. She believes this can help to normalise the experience and to reduce the shame that these women (and men) can feel. In particular, she believes groups can provide a space to "spill long-held secrets and information" that she says can often feel too precious to share with those who do not "get it". Below, she talks about her most recent group and how the participants' own experiences can sometimes help others to 're-frame' a pathway they had previously dismissed.

> I started these groups because none existed when I was on my own infertility journey. I longed for at least one person with whom I could share my ups and downs. It's important, in my view, that the group welcomes women at all stages of their fertility journey, wherever that

may be. Experience has shown that the diversity of the participants, in terms of their various stages of treatment or consideration of treatment, forms the foundation for a rich body of exchange between the participants. As the facilitator, this is what I try to encourage. First, a basis of trust and understanding needs to be established. Often, with this client group, it can happen quite quickly. These women can have a strong bond of identification when each member realises she is in a safe space with others who empathise and understand due to their similar experiences. These women do not want platitudes and sympathy.

Contracting is vital within fertility support group work. This allows the group to consider its own needs for safety, security, and confidentiality. Often, contracting includes discussion and agreement about regular attendance, and no matter how upset someone becomes, the contract is that they will stay with the group, muted if they wish. This is to help them to feel less alone.

In several of my groups, I have had one or two women become pregnant during the group being run. This needs to be discussed at the beginning, during the contracting phase. In one particular group, all had agreed that they would bring their honest and true feelings about the pregnancies, as and when they occurred, even if those feelings were jealousy, envy, and anger. What I wanted was for the women to hear the message that they could bring their whole selves to the group and show it, even the parts they felt were unacceptable.

I recall one participant in her early thirties sharing how devastated she was because her two best friends were pregnant at the same time, and she had just experienced her third failed IVF treatment. She expressed her deep sense of jealousy and anger while also sharing how guilty she felt for feeling this towards women whom she cared for deeply. Often, the shame is twofold: one part is saying, "I cannot have a baby naturally", and the other part is saying, "How can I feel such animosity towards those I love?" Having a space to express these feelings was so important for her. I watched as every head on the screen was nodding in unison. We had all been there too.

Another participant, in her early forties, was facing the reality of repeated IVF failure, with doctors telling her that her best bet was to move to using a donor egg from a younger woman. She shared often about her internal struggles related to letting go of her own eggs, even though she knew they would not viably help her get pregnant. One week, an older participant shared how she now wished she had moved to donor egg and not lost so many years in a state of paralysis, hoping her egg quality would improve when it clearly would not. The first participant was visibly moved by what was shared and said so. In the next week's session, she talked about how deeply impacted she had been by the older woman's story. Several weeks later, she moved on to a clinic to begin her process of IVF using a donor egg.

When reflecting on what they got out of the group work, most participants mention the sense of belonging and identification they feel with other women going through similar processes. This alleviates the loneliness and sense of isolation that comes from making the IVF journey on your own.

The Value of Group Work in the Perinatal

I have chosen to give Valeria Villa the last words in this chapter. She is a TA therapist working with parents and those transitioning into the perinatal period and is so passionate about group work. She has led many different types of parenting groups, such as cross-cultural, baby loss and support groups for therapists who are also parents.

Valeria highlights the value that comes from new mothers coming together as parents in a group, but also the role these women can play in helping to build and form their 'new' Parent ego states, both individually and together as a collective. She also highlights what she sees as the social responsibility of the TA community towards parents, and towards members who are parents:

As a parallel process, new mothers (and new fathers) may feel like newborns (newborn parents) and may connect with other new parents from their inner Child. Because of this, they may disconnect or dissociate from their Parent ego state (for example, from their values, and their life choices, due to confusion, inexperience, and overwhelm). The reality of being in a group can support their Adult to be more present and therefore create more clarity in their Parent ego state. This is of particular value as a support for them to be more equipped to parent.

Another aspect of group work is connected to the silencing phenomenon. For me, there is the political value – in terms of the social responsibility of TA and TA practitioners – to support parents in coming together as a louder voice. There is a responsibility also within the therapeutic community to address this silencing, which I see as 'matricide', where the mother (and mothers) are 'killed off' within our community. There is a responsibility for the therapeutic community to address this both within the TA community, and this would be possible through group work, too.

Conclusion

The aim of this chapter was to show how many possibilities there are to work with all sorts of different themes in TA perinatal psychotherapy groups. Trainees I supervise often say they cannot think of a type of group they could run, yet there are literally hundreds of different topics in the perinatal period.

Perinatal groups need to be carefully thought through and contracted for, particularly for flexibility, around permeability and how the group may be able to cope with changes in some of the members, such as those becoming pregnant. Silencing and shame are inevitable within group work and must be acknowledged. Yet, these types of groups can be powerful and help demystify and de-confuse the parenting process in a space with those who have had similar experiences. They can also give space to those who are marginalised and alienated to speak up, become visible and be heard. Within the groups, participants can experience new and different ways of exploring becoming parents, the pregnancy process, birth and parenting, as each of the members will do it their own particular way. This difference in parenting possibilities may not have been accessible or visible before the group experience, and may go a long way to reassure parents that their way may be the right way for them, even if it is not the right way for others.

11

LOSING A SENSE OF SELF
Fathers and Partners

Written in collaboration with Oliver Hunt

Fathers and non-birthing partners, including adoptive and foster parents, co-mothers and step-parents, deserve their own book. To give them a voice within this one, we want to highlight the difficulties this group of parents can experience and offer some thoughts and reflections on how transactional analytic theory can support them. We aim to focus on some of the most common difficulties these groups of parents can experience, particularly the loss of sense of self.

First, a brief explanation of why we are writing this together. Both of us have a passion for working in the maternal and paternal fields. As a clinician, Oliver works with mothers, fathers and parents, in group, individual and couple settings. His work is similar and yet different to Emma's. We agree that we can be critiqued for offering normative voices of a woman and a man. We are also conscious of a real pull to our respective stereotypical societal 'roles' in our collaboration. In fact, we found ourselves falling into this trap when we first began writing. Emma wrote the bulk of the chapter (the woman doing all the work, perhaps) and Oliver contributed discreet paragraphs but overall deferred to Emma ("good old dad", offering a few sage suggestions on bringing up the 'baby' but remaining outside the actual work). Just as this pattern does not work for many couples, so the chapter felt disjointed, and it was only when we noticed and articulated the parallel process that we found a new direction and a genuine collaborative voice.

We also need to highlight immediately that we are not a couple. We are two psychotherapists with a passion to support parents, in whatever form, in raising the next generations. We both have lived experience of the lack of support offered in the UK. And we both recognise systemic failure in maternal and parental support throughout the world and the negative impact this can have on family life.

Parenting works best as a joint task, with everyone benefiting from some support. Being a single parent is really tough. Sharing the parenting experience can ease the burden of care financially, socially, psychologically and physically. Two parents raising a child also offers difference and diversity, both vitally important for the child to experience. This is not only about

DOI: 10.4324/9781003365822-11

gender, but in thoughts, opinions, fears, perspectives, desires, observations, social attributes, and all manner of things. Children need this diversity to develop their creativity, uniqueness, resilience, innovation, and their social and psychological tolerance. We also know the critical importance of offering a safe and secure environment to infants and children, and the difference this has on the child's ability to feel safe, secure, attached and regulated. Without this, as stated earlier in this book, it is difficult for a child to grow into a healthy functioning adult, with emotional intelligence and self-regulation.

We hope that writing this chapter in collaboration will bring it alive and help it to remain real. We are both sensitive to what we perceive as a polarisation in many countries and societies, in which man seems to be pitched against woman. This binary thinking feels like a regression in the system, and we seriously question the motives behind this polarisation and wonder about the worrying growth in misogyny we see, and the consequences this may have on future generations and family life.

Parents can identify in many different ways. We want to open up dialogue towards empowering and honouring all expressions of gender and sexuality and all types of parents and their partners. Although we write from our heterosexual experience, as parents and as therapists, we aim to be as inclusive as possible, and to understand we are bound by our limitations. We believe it is crucial to leave dialogue open, curious and honest with good intentions so that we can all learn from experiences of difference, fluidity and all of life's expressions of gender and parenting. The terms father and partner are used throughout to be expansive and to capture all these terms might mean. For example, they might not mean male or paternal and might not be situated in men and might include co-mothers, co-fathers, and step-parents. We aim not to exclude anyone in this chapter; however, we also understand that, despite the best of intentions, we will. We also acknowledge that we both approach our work from a UK-based, Western perspective, so although we strive to consider other cultures, inevitably we are limited by our own frames of reference.

We hope this chapter enlivens the difficulties befalling fathers and partners. More than anything, this is an exploration of what we all can do to change the support available for parents, couples and families and to make a difference to children's lives.

Navigating the Pathway to Parenthood

Like mothers, fathers and partners can also struggle in their earliest transitions to parenthood, and when difficulties arise, psychotherapy can help them resource themselves to prepare for this shift in their role and mitigate some of these struggles. It can be useful to explore ambivalence and fear of becoming a parent and the new responsibilities that are arising. This fear is often about the economic and psychological costs of rearing a child and employment pressures. It can also be fear of repeating past neglectful or harmful patterns.

For many years the mental health of fathers and partners was neglected and overlooked. Yet they experience perinatal mental illness too, although often in different ways to women. Their symptoms are more likely to be anger, hyperactive behaviour, irritability and lower impulse control (O'Brien et al., 2017; Williamson, 1987; Winkler, Pjrek & Kasper, 2005). However, little research has occurred on the mental illness of fathers and partners. What research there is has been aimed at fathers rather than being inclusive of all types of parents and partners. We thought it would be more helpful to focus on areas common to all partners, particularly the 'paternal' role and how it is experienced within a family. Exploring the benefits of this role can facilitate parental communication and negotiation rather than reverting to inherited script patterns. Included in this could be an exploration of what masculinity offers and how it can hinder the dyad.

Areas for discussion can be all manner of things: cultural scripting, finding a role, common parental fears, sex and intimacy, the impact of parental experiences such as artificial reproductive techniques (ART) and in vitro fertilisation (IVF), miscarriage, vicarious trauma and the diverse cultural myths that abound. In particular, navigating and negotiating the partner's role, who does what, who cares for whom, and why, often such a sticky area between a couple, and helping partners find some options for navigating this, particularly when there is a sense of blame and shame due to difficulties with conception. Exploring these can help to mitigate their power. The focus is on delving into the relationship between the parents, from the father's and partner's angle, to engender support.

The Evolving Nature of Parenting

The father's or partner's role in co-raising their infants from birth through to adulthood has been downplayed, ignored or taboo in many societies until relatively recently. However, there is a growing recognition that, due to economic pressures, families throughout the world cannot survive without both parents working. Yet, there has been a huge lack of division in care, with gender inequalities occurring both inside and outside the home. Reports such as *The State of the World's Fathers* (Van der Gaag et al., 2019) help to push for change in social and gender norms as a move towards greater equality, and promote changes in laws and policies worldwide. These are the first steps towards fathers and partners stepping up into the caregiving role. Evidence shows that sharing of care can improve fathers' mental health and well-being, increase job satisfaction, enhance work–family life, and lead to less work–family conflict (Chung, 2021; Ladge et al., 2015).

Even though more fathers and partners throughout the world are choosing to play a greater role in sharing the care of their children, such as in the US (Chesley, 2011; Solomon, 2017), Belgium (Merla, 2008), Canada (Shafer & Renick, 2020), Norway (Brandth & Kvande, 2016) and the UK (Chung et al., 2020), there is nowhere near the equality needed in caregiving, particularly to infants and young children. This is despite research showing that 85% of fathers from Argentina, Brazil, Canada, Japan, the US, the UK and the Netherlands say they "would be willing to do anything to be very involved in caring for their new child" (van der Gaag et al., 2019, p. 47).

The COVID-19 pandemic influenced fathers and partners to take on more of the caregiving almost certainly by having to remain at home with their partner and children, due to the closing of schools and childcare facilities (Carlson, Petts & Pepin, 2020; Chung et al., 2020; Craig & Churchill, 2020). However, there still seems to be an ongoing systemic failure to recognise that caregiving is a societal responsibility and that fathers and partners also need help and support.

Fathers and male partners sharing in the care, or who are the predominant carer, can feel isolated and marginalised in daytime parenting spaces. This is a systemic problem that is downplayed, yet has an impact on those fathers who want to be involved in their children's lives. Fathers and partners need to be included in the entirety of pregnancy and post-birth as part of the ritual of their transition into parenthood. This inclusion must be a natural part of medical practice and within society, with a paradigm shift towards it being abnormal for them not to be.

The transition to becoming a parent is challenging for fathers and partners, bringing exhaustion, confusion, loneliness, and feeling trapped within their new role (Rowe, Holton & Fisher, 2013). In fact, expectant fathers and partners can experience Couvade syndrome – physical symptoms, most commonly in the first and third trimester of the pregnancy, which are inexplicable such as weight gain, diarrhoea, stomach cramps, and indigestion that may be caused by underlying heightened anxiety and difficulties in transitioning into father/parenthood. Whereas previously, there has not been much in the way of research into the comorbidity of couples' mood disorders, there is now some evidence that both parents can experience perinatal mood disorders at the same time, with estimates of around 3.18% of parental couples experiencing low mood concurrently (Smythe, Petersen & Schartau, 2022). Clearly, this will impact the infant/child in some way, although I could find no research yet about what that impact might be.

No matter how hard a couple prepare for becoming parents, it will never be entirely as predicted and both parents can lose a sense of self in this transition. Although it seems obvious, sometimes it is quite a shock when fathers and partners feel overlooked and neglected, marginalised even after a highly traumatic birth experience. Within the last 40 or 50 years, fathers and partners have become more actively involved in the birth process, which is a positive factor for the mother's well-being and helps to enhance coping abilities for the couple. Notwithstanding, many still say they feel like a spare part or feel in the way, particularly during a medical birth.

Yet, fathers and partners are a crucial and vital support network, and their mental health needs to be resilient enough so they can perform their role and bond with their child, particularly now, as there seems to be a cultural shift in the US and in many European countries towards a more significant role and involvement in child rearing from partners and fathers. The American Psychological Association (APA) draw attention to this change and how it helps to promote a child's development, both socially and emotionally (APA, 2009). If the mother is experiencing maternal disturbance and distress, the father or partner's role becomes paramount, acting as a buffer between the impact of the mother's condition on the infant and any child development issues. They are also a support and advocate for the mother, which can be vital if the mother is unable or not well enough to advocate for herself.

Questions to explore:

What is the partner coming for?

What do they actually want to achieve in therapy?

What is going under the radar – what cannot be said by the partner or between the couple?

How is the partner envisaging parenthood, if the baby has not yet arrived, or if the couple are experiencing IVF or ART?

Is there some ambivalence about becoming a parent?

Do they understand and know what they want in their role as a parent? Has this been explored and discussed?

How do they feel at the prospect of becoming a parent? Do they feel like an equal partner in the process or that it's something happening to them?

What are their deep fears – are they afraid they won't know how to do it?

Often, fathers or partners try hard to be the best they can for their partner and child but struggle to know how to help. Several things that have become apparent for us in writing this chapter is the lack of natural inclusion of fathers and partners within the pregnancy and parental journey, particularly among medical staff but also within society. Why are fathers and partners still being excluded and marginalised in this way? Why do men still report feeling out of place in daytime caring environments, to the extent they choose to avoid them in favour of more solitary activities? Even though they have been somewhat welcome in the birthing room for four decades or so, this is not always the case with routine examinations, or medical emergencies around the mother and infant, with reports of men feeling excluded, unwanted, an imposter, a nuisance or a spare part (by the medical staff, not the mother). This, despite best practice in medical systems, according to the WHO and UN, is to include the father/partner.

Research on Fathers

The incidence of perinatal depression and anxiety is between 5% (Mazza et al., 2022) and 10–15% in fathers (Cameron et al., 2016; Leach et al., 2016; Paulson & Bazemore, 2010). Maternal depression is a common risk factor for paternal perinatal depression and anxiety (Chhabra, Li & McDermott, 2022), and there seems to be a possible interconnection of symptomatology between parents (Cameron et al., 2016; Figueiredo et al., 2018). There is virtually no research on partners as yet.

Other risk factors are low income (Bergström, 2013), substance abuse (Bronte-Tinkew et al., 2007) and a history of psychiatric illness (Ramchandani et al., 2005). One strong predictor of postnatal anxiety and depression in fathers is attachment anxiety (Psouni, Frisk & Brocki, 2021). Partners can also experience post-traumatic stress due to witnessing a particularly traumatic birth, and partners are also known to be at greater risk of suicide within this period (Darwin et al., 2021). Darwin et al. also draw attention to the increased risk for co-mothers and trans and gender-diverse parents, particularly noting the "distinct challenges" of stigma, marginalisation, ART, and a lack of legal recognition as parents (Darwin et al., 2021) in some countries, Italy for example, although there is a real lack of research about this. Good quality screening tools that help identify partners at risk of mental health difficulties are needed worldwide. There is also some evidence that fathers/partners feel that health professionals overlook their mental health needs (Daniels, Arden-Close & Mayers, 2020; Darwin et al., 2017; Mayers et al., 2020; Rominov et al., 2018). Depression and anxiety in fathers and partners may be expressed in different ways to maternal depression, such as with increases in anger, irritability and withdrawal (Cochran & Rabinowitz, 2003), causing difficulties in diagnosis (Singley & Edwards, 2015).

It is also known that poor postnatal mental health in fathers and partners can have a significant impact on the infant (Chhabra et al., 2022), causing difficulties such as child behavioural problems at three and a half years of age (Ramchandani et al., 2005) and at seven years of age (Ramchandani et al., 2008). The incidence of paternal perinatal mood disorders is also likely to have an economic impact on mental health services (Edoka, Petrou & Ramchandani, 2011).

Fathers are even less willing to speak about and seek help for their mental health than mothers, and often view psychotherapy negatively, with a reluctance to remain in treatment (Addis & Mahalik, 2003; Mansfield, Addis & Mahalik, 2003; Primack et al., 2010). Misinterpretation can occur, particularly when considering the added stress of having a new baby with the pressure and fatigue. Many men struggle with little or no support network and can be reliant on their partners for this support. When the mother is already struggling and possibly preoccupied with her new role, this support is often

not as forthcoming as it might have been prior, causing some men to feel isolated and alone, which can lead to them adopting negative coping strategies
such as resorting to alcohol and drug-taking, and a preoccupation towards
working.

Interestingly, the role of parenthood is more likely to be idealised by men
(Condon, Boyce & Corkindale, 2004). Thus, some men can find the inevitable
rupture of the idealised parent particularly painful.

Cultural Scripting: Masculinity

Men state they feel stigma around seeking treatment for perinatal anxiety
and depression, mainly due to societal expectations of the role men should
or should not play in their children's lives, a role which has been centuries in
the making. One helpful area and essential to explore is masculinity, particularly now when discussions abound around toxic masculinity. In the US, for
example, the APA published *Guidelines for Psychological Practice with Boys
and Men* to try to address some of the difficulties men and boys are experiencing and to highlight how masculinity is "psychologically harmful" and
"traditional masculinity—marked by stoicism, competitiveness, dominance
and aggression—is, on the whole, harmful" (APA, 2018).

How can the masculine norms of stoicism and self-reliance be confronted
when some men see entering therapy as going against their need to be strong,
wearing their strength as a badge of honour? The difficulty with this is that
men and partners do experience depression, trauma and anxiety in the perinatal period, and some studies are showing that adding in panic disorder
and acute adjustment disorder with anxiety can raise the incidence to 100%
(Matthey et al., 2003).

It would be easy to assume that the drivers and injunctions of masculinity
are the Be Strong/Don't Feel matrix. This certainly can be true, with the partner assuming the need to be strong enough to cope for the family. Research
by Yousaf, Popat and Hunter (2015) shows the reluctance men have to seek
out help for mental health difficulties. The consequence of this might mean a
need to cut off from feelings to remain strong or perhaps a denial of self-care
behaviours.

In therapy, there can be an expectation that the father/partner will show
up and be vulnerable. Yet, how easy is this? Could therapists place too much
pressure on showing vulnerability? If men like to think of themselves as the
ones to solve problems, how easy is it for them to recognise and face up to
changes such as prolonged sadness, stress, loss of independence, opioid or
alcohol dependence, a change in libido or difficulties with memory loss? The
APA highlight the need for clinicians to know their own biases and to know
the dominant masculine ideals in their cultures, subcultures and ethnic groups
(APA, 2019).

Exploring masculinity:

How do you feel about yourself as a man?
How do you feel about who you are as a parent?
What does vulnerability mean to you?
What does the term masculinity mean to you?
What were the messages growing up about masculinity?
Who was your role model of male behaviour?
Where do aggression and anger fit in, and are they acceptable emotions?
What about anxiety? Do you feel anxious of your role as a parent?
What about distance and aloofness, being there but yet not there?
What is the split between earning money and child rearing? Whose role
   is which?
What do you think about your role as caregiver?
Who does the patriarchy serve?

The two things that seem to afflict many men, regardless of who they are, where they live, and the culture they grew up in, are that men seldom like to ask for help, and many men struggle to talk about their feelings. What is it about speaking about emotions that puts men off? Is it that vulnerability can be conflated with weakness – a fear of letting others in and diminishing the father's view of themselves as strong? Minikin's work on alienation (2018, 2021a, 2021b) is helpful in this regard and clarifies the damage of masculine stereotyping. To expect men to be up front with their feelings from the outset of therapy requires a level of bravery that may be too much for some. Perhaps a way into feelings can be to focus on accessible psychoeducational concepts, such as the Drama Triangle and driver behaviour. As a generalisation, men's 'open door' of contact (Ware, 1983) often appears to be thinking, so providing ideas and diagrams that can be understood and discussed intellectually can lead later to reflections about feelings and behaviour.

Men seem to respond well to the idea of the winner's triangle as a way to find a balance between what might be seen as masculine potency and feminine responsiveness and vulnerability. We (Emma and Oliver) have been exploring and debating what seems to be a solution-focused stereotyping of men. Is this truly part of a man's makeup? Part of the need for a man to be the hunter–gatherer of the past, solution-focused on finding food and protecting their families? Or is it a part of a socially constructed masculinity that has become a stereotype-casting of men? Is this even actually about gender, or is this cultural scripting, and how might we begin to differentiate these elements? What is true in the numerous different cultures?

A gulf often seems to exist between intention and impact regarding how a man's words affect his partner. In attempting to fix a problem or find a solution, men might not notice the implied criticism in their words or when the partner wants their feelings acknowledged rather than the problem to be solved. Self-disclosure, when used with discretion, can be a powerful tool in challenging the cultural script around masculinity. If a male therapist demonstrates that it is okay to be vulnerable and to feel emotion, this can help to decontaminate inherited beliefs, particularly around male authority figures. Two men who can experience emotion together can offer a profound rewriting of script.

Some considerations when exploring script are the intergenerational, epigenetic experience, the client's experience of the 'Father' archetype when growing up (nurturing, punishing, absent?). Exploring the father's/partner's experience when young, encouraging them to ask questions of older family members, for example, and being curious about the transgenerational inherited scripting can unlock possible familial impasses that may be felt at some level but seem non-narratable. It is still only a couple of generations from the Second World War's colossal societal and personal trauma, and older clients might even have been born or in the womb during the conflict. Did our client have a father or grandfather who fought in the war, and what was the effect of that experience on him and then on his offspring? How has this shaped his sons and daughters and their offspring? Was his father or grandfather perhaps a part of the trauma of the First World War as well? Perhaps the cultural norm of men not talking about their feelings was highlighted by the effect of post-traumatic stress, protecting themselves by staying emotionally distant from their children and reinforcing the societal norm of Be Strong/Don't Feel.

For a stereotypical European man, there might seem to be a sense of "I'm okay, You are not" defence, particularly when talking about maternal distress, that the problem is situated in the mother. What is essential is to find a way to challenge this view within the therapeutic domain in a non-shaming way. This is not necessarily easy when what may be seen within therapy is the patriarchal defence of "I'm not the problem here; it is all hers as she is the one who has 'gone through' this and has her hormones raging". However, as pointed out earlier in this book, women may take the blame in society due to the assumptions and generalisations prevalent in a patriarchal society. Let's briefly explore this view of patriarchy, consider how it does not serve society, and attempt to bring freshness to this long-lived trope.

Finding a Role: "Who Am I Now?"

A dichotomy seems to continue to exist, which is one with patriarchal foundations: the tension between the 'father figure' and the power this figure holds within the family, and the perpetuated absence of and marginalisation of the father from family life due to the outdated and outmoded stereotypical view that parenting is particularly and exclusively a female activity. This dichotomy discounts and negates the importance of the father in an infant's life. Thankfully, more writers are challenging dad stereotypes, and research findings from neuroscience, genetics and psychology are being published on just how important the father is in the life of their infant (Machin, 2018) and how this positively impacts the mental health of the child as they grow up (Smyth & Russell, 2021). Many studies show how the father's involvement correlates with the child's academic achievement (Flouri & Buchanan, 2003) and the positive effects of having an involved father (Institute for Research on Poverty, 2020).

So how can we help fathers/partners to find their new role, to question and challenge them in a way that opens dialogue and exploration and allows them to feel in control of who they are becoming and, indeed, who they want to be as a parent? Is this new persona someone who will model parenting in a positive way? Is this a figure who is the opposite of their parents and who offers perhaps something novel, yearned for, offers hope of a different experience?

As shown earlier, change has occurred within many family structures, and many men now assume the role of caregiver and are more deeply involved with the upbringing of their children. For example, in the developed world, Moran et al. (2021) report that up to 96% of all fathers are present at the birth of their child. Men are also increasingly coming for one-to-one therapy for many reasons, one of which may be to deal with their paternal deficits. Transitioning from being fathered to becoming a father can highlight difficulties with their father figure. Yet, fathers are a central part of their children's lives and help with their emotional well-being, social interactions and educational achievements (O'Dwyer, 2017).

However, there is a decline in the number of children who live with their biological fathers, particularly with the increase in divorce, the decline in marriage, and the growth in children born to parents who are not in a stable partnership. How do we enable these parents to participate in their children's lives and establish a successful co-parenting relationship? Can the TA community be a part of the growing consensus and body of evidence that promotes father's involvement and adds to this with its own model of fatherhood and of the paternal that honours the unique value a father offers their child, particularly as Machin (2018) points out, in the way that fathers orientate their infants outward towards the world?

Resourcing Fathers and Partners

A group setting can be a powerful way of providing space for men to speak about their experiences or fears around parenthood. Offering a space for men to be vulnerable and talk about their feelings may feel like going against the patriarchal cultural scripting of the need to be as strong as possible, and some men may feel it is simply weird to talk about their feelings. This is useful to consider when setting up a group. Focusing on problem-solving and facilitating support of a partner struggling with perinatal mental illness may be more inviting for a man. Such groups often attract the woman who responds to the advertisement, saying what a great idea it is and how many men would benefit. Sadly, only a few men get in touch and come. What can attract men to join such a group? What puts men off?

Communication and Couples Work

This book has a whole chapter on couples work (see Chapter 9). However, it is important to acknowledge couples work here, too, as communication within a couple who are parenting is vital. In couples work, it can often be one person who gets in touch. This can lead to a game invitation from the outset, and looking for any hook into a game setup is important. This can be a game of 'ganging up' on either the father/partner (showing up is harder) or equally against the woman, who may be seen as overreacting or even hysterical by her partner.

The birth of an infant tends to hijack the space and time a couple used to have pre-children, which can lead to assumptions about many aspects of parenting which may go unspoken. When there are cultural differences, these can appear suddenly, with a sense of "I didn't know you felt that way" or perhaps a family expectation around the infant. This may lead to resentment and a hierarchy of suffering, the sense that the mother is the focus, sidelining and discounting the partner's experience. Many fathers speak of feeling a sense of "I shouldn't be complaining", particularly if the birth was traumatic. The partner may then remain silent about how challenging their experience was because they believe their partner cannot and should not hear it. Self-silencing can happen for the father/partner too.

It can be helpful to remind couples of the need for space for themselves to be an adult and a parent, and to this end, using the metaphor of putting their oxygen mask on before they can help others is worthwhile. When things become overwhelming, how do they react? Is it to distance themselves from the difficulty or to be consumed by the other's needs and neglect themselves? How does a couple communicate and negotiate about what both need to feel okay? Parental guilt can take many forms but can be avoided by honest communication between partners. There are many aspects to be negotiated within a couple, such as work patterns within and outside the family, cultural elements, and how to make the best choices for the family together, rather than assuming we know who does what, who earns what, and who cares for whom.

The best time for a couple to wrestle with these difficult conversations is during pre-conception, as stated earlier. Does there need to be a paradigm shift in parenting so that young couples are encouraged to have these discussions before the infant arrives or, even more preferably, before conception? Facilitating these communications offers an opportunity for couples to talk about what they both assume about parenting and their expectations around becoming parents together. It is surprising that these communications are not obligatory for such a huge, lifelong commitment as having children. It is all too common for communication to break down, leading to conflict and shame.

It is useful to open up space within relationships to explore complex and sometimes embarrassing elements: fear of the inevitable changes in the relationship with our partner; how to keep enough of what is important between the couple while also devoting themselves to their children; hormonal fluctuations some women experience postpartum; desire or lack of desire with the consequent feelings of rejection; what can go under the radar when it comes to sex; what can happen if there has been physical trauma during birth; helping the father/partner think about what it might be like for the mother to have a tiny person utterly dependent on her body to fulfil its survival needs and the jealousy this can bring, feeling pushed out perhaps, where it can feel like the baby is the only thing the mother is interested in at that time. Psychotherapy can really help the father/partner to understand how reliant the infant is on the mother, and that she needs to be focused on the infant's needs and to explore what the impact might be on the relationship and how the father may be able to offer support and care in the early weeks and months when the mother is absorbed with her infant. The overwhelming nature of this dependency might mean that the last thing she wants is demands from someone else to touch her.

Miscarriage, Stillbirth, IVF: Processing Grief

How does a partner experience loss? It would be easy to assume that the partner won't experience miscarriage as a loss, or at least not the same loss as the mother. What's more, when listening to mothers and partners, there is a continued invitation to gloss over and discount their experience at the level of existence, with comments like "it wasn't a real baby", "get pregnant again", "get over it, plenty more time". If the mother is being told to discount her pregnancy, then the expectation for the partner to get over it is even greater. What space is there for the partner to experience grief? Of course, we all experience grief differently; some can process the miscarriage and seem to move on much quicker than others, and this will very much depend on our own coping strategies and resilience. Yet scars get left behind. When partners come into therapy, they often don't come to process grief directly. They can come for a multitude of reasons. Opening up space for whatever they bring, helping them to acknowledge how these difficulties have impacted them and giving permission to speak about the impact on them can offer a release and relief in how to dialogue about this.

A loss in pregnancy, or a difficulty with fertility, can put enormous strain on a partnership, with blame and shame between partners. This is particularly true if one person is singled out as the contributory factor: perhaps their eggs are not developing well, they are going through the menopause much earlier than normal, or they have a low sperm count. Is it easier to blame yourself or the other rather than to feel the tragedy and grieve for it? Is this a masculine trope, the idea that men need to be the strong ones and should not show their feelings? What happens to them when they do this? How does this impact their sense of self, the way they identify themselves in the partnership? It can be helpful to encourage the partner to identify their favoured positions on the OK Corral. Thinking this through with them and helping them to see the possible outcome of their position, the added burden this can place on the relationship. Assisting the partner in seeing their role in the relationship strain can be helpful and may unlock any impasse. When becoming a father, how much of our expectations are governed by our own experiences, either conforming and repeating our script or rebelling and deciding to do something different?

Vicarious Trauma and Post-traumatic Stress

Fathers and partners can experience birth trauma from witnessing their wife/partner endure a particularly difficult or gruelling labour or the death of the mother or infant during labour and birth. When experiencing this type of trauma, fathers/partners often speak of feeling powerless and unable to help their partner or even advocate for her, stating a sense of being pushed aside by the medical profession. Little attention has been paid to birth trauma within the mother, and even less attention is given to vicarious trauma in the father or partner. Vicarious trauma is the exposure to a traumatic event in which the person witnessing believes injury or death is occurring due to the medical intervention of health professionals. Witnessing such an event can have a significant impact, with an apparent mirroring of the mother's response in the witness, including experiencing post-traumatic stress disorder (Iles, Slade & Spiby, 2011). Unfortunately, little attention is paid to the father or partner, leading them to feel isolated and abandoned. One coping strategy is simply not talking about the event, minimising the distress and calling it "unjustified" (Daniels et al., 2020). Some studies have shown the lack of information received by fathers in the birth process was problematic, with men stating the need to be informed rather than a need to be involved (Eggermont et al., 2017). For some, a lack of control can be the most terrifying part (Daniels et al., 2020), with long-term effects on happiness, the sense of self (particularly manhood), and the consequent impact this had on their long-term relationships.

Outside the Heteronormative Dyad

In considering parenting and relationships, we acknowledge that it can be easy to focus on the heterosexual norm. This chapter has largely explored the experiences of men and fathers, but we also want to give space and a voice to the increasing number of couples who are not falling into the traditional parenting dyad. Yet there is so little research to do this. What is it like to adopt or have a surrogate baby from within a same-sex relationship? What is it like for co-mothers if one carries a baby through pregnancy? Does the other then donate their egg? If fathers tend to feel isolated within parenting circles, what prejudices might co-fathers encounter every day that add to the already heavy burden of parenthood? What sort of prejudice do single-sex couples experience throughout their daily life?

Client Vignette: Ravi

Ravi is a 42-year-old British Indian man whose parents emigrated from India in the 1970s. He and his wife went through two courses of IVF before a successful pregnancy, and their daughter is now three. Ravi initially came to therapy looking for help with a sense of burnout and problems with sleeping, and gradually it emerged how this was linked to his cultural and familial expectations of masculinity and fatherhood.

Like many second-generation immigrants, Ravi's experience was of an environment that expected men to work hard to provide for their families. His father worked six days a week plus whatever overtime he could find and was emotionally unavailable for his family. He had a clearly defined role of 'provider', while Ravi's mother looked after the children. As the youngest of three, Ravi had the pressure of trying to live up to the achievements of his high-flying older siblings, succumbing to the belief that he was stupid because he found school difficult. His father would become angry and threatening whenever Ravi came home with a report that did not live up to his expectations, and Ravi learned how to stay hidden at school and home, living in fear of the consequences of being seen. His father was also violent towards his mother, so she focused on staying safe by keeping him happy rather than providing emotional support for the children; the whole family "walked on eggshells".

A crucial aspect of therapy sessions was exploring Ravi's desires and experiences around fatherhood. He wanted to be different from his own father and have a close connection with his daughter, but he did not know how. He found that at weekends he would make excuses to go and work at his home office rather than be with his family. Exploring this impasse at a cognitive level did not improve things – he might go away with a plan to change the dynamic but come back saying, "I couldn't do it, I just needed to work". Over time we discovered further layers to this: there was a Type II impasse around a sense of fear, and he became emotional when he realised that he did not know how to play with his daughter, as no one had ever played with him. He was afraid of the part of himself that might end up being like his father. Further work explored a deep sense of bodily neglect that played out through food; he seemed cut off from his body and often would ignore impulses such as hunger, fuelled by an existential sense of despair – "What's the point?".

Something of Ravi's early experience of neglect and fear seemed to have been introjected into a sense of self as "not enough", which he attempted to counteract by following the masculine cultural script of hard work. When I asked, "What would be enough?" his answer was "I don't know". The lack of an internalised Nurturing Parent played out in not looking after himself and not knowing how to be with his daughter in the way he wanted.

As a male therapist, I felt a pull also to Try Hard in our sessions, and it was very tempting to suggest cognitive solutions myself. Instead, I tried to stay attuned to his experience and provide something of the unconditional positive regard that he lacked in his early days. One day he came in and announced, "Something feels different. I spent the weekend with the family, and while part of me kept saying, 'You should go and work', I managed to ignore it". By uncovering his masculine cultural script and providing space for his vulnerable self to feel accepted, Ravi could begin to decide what sort of father *he* wanted to be.

Working with Ravi helped me to reflect on gender roles across different cultures, and how different pressures can lead to a similar result: the tendency in men of both British and Indian heritage to Be Strong and stay cut off from their emotions. Using empathic confrontation (Clark, 1991) to challenge the status quo, and finding a space where a therapeutic relationship between two men could acknowledge and tolerate emotion, has led to a gradual shift in his sense of self.

Conclusion

This clinical example leads back to where we began the chapter: that fathers and partners can lose their sense of self in their parental role, be it from an inability to connect emotionally, or a desire to do things so differently they lose focus on what they need; from a desire to conform to or rebel against a cultural script, or discover that they have never known who they truly are. In a sense, the chapter feels like it has asked more questions than supplied answers, perhaps mirroring the therapeutic process itself. By enquiring into fathers' and partners' experiences, allowing space for their personal truth to emerge, we can help provide an environment for them to rediscover that sense of self, and become the parents they aspire to be.

12

COMPLEX PRESENTATIONS, DISTURBANCE AND SELF-CARE

I highlighted the most common perinatal presentations in Chapter 3. In this chapter, I want to emphasise some of the more complex presentations. This is to draw attention to the thorny intricacies of some perinatal work, which has the capacity to draw the psychotherapist into deep, transferential processes. This can feel overwhelming, frightening and engulfing and also risk therapist burnout. I continue to be curious, nosey even, about why, with some clients, the work can feel so knotty and demanding, the client really getting under my skin, poking and prodding me at a level I didn't know existed. Cornell and Landaiche speak about the reluctance we may have to experience the disturbances of our client. Yet, with complex perinatal presentations, disturbance is an inevitability. Some clients evoke feelings in us that are agitating at the very least, and can be downright terrifying at the worst. How do we mitigate against this disturbance?

Cornell and Landaiche speak of those aspects in our work as psychotherapists that disturb us.

> The contact we can make with states of self that do not readily lend themselves to words or diagrams, many of us are reluctant to experience the disturbances our clients bring to and evoke in us. Yet such disturbances seem an inevitable consequence of the intimacy that develops in every therapeutic and consulting relationship. The very nature of such close contact between any two or more human beings is bound to affect us at levels that operate outside of consciousness and that inform our most fundamental patterns of relating. As a result, we may discover ourselves and our working relationships stalled in habitual ways of being, often accompanied by feelings of frustration, anger, and a sense of inadequacy. Once our work has become so maddeningly stuck, how do we find our way back to productive engagement?
>
> (2006, p. 197)

In Chapter 8 on creativity I offered some thoughts on addressing the stuckness in maternal and perinatal work. In this chapter, I want to highlight the

DOI: 10.4324/9781003365822-12

types of perinatal presentations that can bring disturbance and emphasise how important it is for psychotherapists to integrate self-care into their everyday practice in order to guard against this disturbance. When working in the maternal sphere, self-care is crucial, as parental protocol and transgenerational mental illness and disturbance are very much part of this work, and the possibility of burnout is high. Perinatal work so often means walking the knife-edge between life and death and joy and utter grief with our clients. Burnout takes a toll on and impairs the mental health and clinical judgement therapists rely on, hampering their ability to work consistently from client to client. Self-care is vital for both client and therapist, particularly with complex perinatal presentations.

Conditions I will highlight are co-parenting a child with high dependency care, disabilities and/or with a terminal diagnosis; parenting with a chronic health condition or disability; postpartum psychosis; severe trauma; and historic mental health disorders such as schizophrenia, or bipolar disorder.

Co-parenting a Child with High Dependency Care, Disabilities and/or with a Terminal Diagnosis

Sadly, around 7 million children die each year worldwide, and estimates suggest around 21 million would benefit from palliative care. Co-parenting a child with high dependency needs, with severe disabilities or with a terminal diagnosis is hugely painful and also intensely emotional and exhausting (Barrett et al., 2023), yet parents somehow still need to fulfil their parenting role. It can mean parents struggle with their mental and physical health as there is an expectation they will assume many different roles for the child, often with little in the way of help – physical, emotional, social, spiritual and medical roles, for example – leaving the parents with little energy, feeling drained or overwhelmed and for some, close to collapse.

Parents often have to make tough decisions about their child's care, which can add to sometimes already complicated family dynamics and struggles. This can be compounded with financial strains due to the significant levels of care the child may require, leaving little time for holding down a job, or the risk of losing their job due to being unable to give work the attention it might need. The parents also may be asked to subject their child to painful procedures or medical care, which goes against the typical role of a parent, to protect their child from pain and discomfort. This can lead to high levels of guilt and fear that this may impact their relationship with the child. It is such a very different role for parents when their expectation was to parent a healthy child into maturity. Yet, they find themselves caring for a child who may well decline and die or who will have significant needs later in life.

There are likely to be difficulties for other children in the family, too, as the sick child may hold a special status in the family. Yet for other children, there is a normal household routine, with rules and chores. This may be perceived as unfair, or that siblings feel neglected by the parents. Family therapy can be helpful if it incorporates everyone and allows siblings to speak up about their experiences of life.

Many of the emotional outcomes of this type of parenting will be similar to other perinatal complications: experiencing anxiety, depressive symptoms, guilt, stress and fear. There are added elements, too, that may become apparent, such as parents with varying degrees of uncertainty and disbelief who may be in denial about their child's health outcome or who feel powerless and angry and experience high levels of grief. For parents of children with a terminal diagnosis, there is also the anticipatory and realised grief of their child's condition. Long-term grief can become problematic and unrelenting for these parents, and there is a real risk of some parents developing PTSD.

I have found it helpful to support the parents to orientate themselves towards their child's pain and distress without it being self-oriented. This sounds simple but is more difficult than it appears. Parents who are struggling may display catastrophic thinking and this can impact the child and increase their own catastrophic thinking. Research from Lynch and Lobo (2012) found that a parent's capacity to catastrophise meant the child was also more likely to catastrophise, which was not helpful for the child's health.

One fundamental difficulty may be mothers experiencing a high level of guilt or a sense that they did something to cause the child to be born with disabilities. This guilt can be so severe that some parents experience dark thoughts about both themselves and the infant and may have high levels of suicidal ideation. As with working with any client with suicidal ideation, the therapist will benefit from having a great deal of supervisory support through this. It may also be necessary to work together with psychiatric teams, if necessary.

My experience of this type of complexity was working with a woman who had wanted to terminate her baby. Unfortunately, she was too far into her pregnancy for this to be an option. Our work was initially challenging during her pregnancy as she was unable to contemplate bonding with her infant before giving birth, as she expressed a high degree of resentment about her situation. As a mother myself, this was difficult to sit with, and I needed to explore my responses in both supervision and therapy. However, post-birth her feelings about her infant began to change, and she was able to bond and attach to her baby. The mother also had a close support network around her and was able to gain help in raising her infant, which meant she was willing to explore and find a way through her original fantasy that life would be a disaster with a child. For me, I found it hard to remain neutral as I found her resentment disturbed me. I don't think I would have been able to work at depth with her if I had not received strong supervisory support.

Helping parents allow enough time for their own emotional well-being with a child with a high level of need can also positively impact the child's well-being (Koch & Jones, 2018). Unsurprisingly, Koch and Jones' research evidence shows that parents who were unable to focus on their own health were less able to cope with their child's needs. For parents struggling with their own self-care, I often use the metaphor of an airplane's oxygen mask and the need for a parent to attend to their own oxygen mask first before helping their child. Many parents are so geared towards their child's health needs that even thinking about their own causes guilt and stress.

There is a similar need for parents to help each other through helping them explore relationship-focused strategies to cope with the difficulties in their family. It is possible to help couples build and maintain their relationships during these difficult times. Many parents find their relationship is so low down the list of priorities that it gets forgotten until it is too late. Sadly, some couples end up splitting apart when they have such difficult family environments (Anchesi et al., 2023). However, this is not necessarily a certainty, and it is useful to reassure couples that if they can find new ways to cope together, it might positively impact their relationship.

Pregnancy, Birth and Parenting with a Disability or Chronic Health Conditions

Chronic illness is now much more common in pregnant mothers and during birth (Admon et al., 2017; Gogoi & Unisa, 2017). Unfortunately, this type of illness can have negative outcomes for some mothers and their infants, such as their illness changing and developing, causing increased stress and new medical needs (Tyer-Viola & Lopez, 2014). With the advances in medicine, many women with chronic health complications are now able to experience pregnancy and birth when they might not have been able to decades ago. Women with multiple sclerosis (MS), for example, used to be told to abstain from pregnancy in the 1920s and 30s. However, it is now known that MS can even go into a temporary period of remission with pregnancy. It can be similar for other diseases too, such as epilepsy and for a few women with diabetes (Kersten et al., 2014). Yet other conditions may not go into remission, such as fibromyalgia (Al-Allaf et al., 2002; Furness et al., 2018; Galvez-Sánchez, Duschek & Reyes Del Paso, 2019). There are many chronic diseases which women can have which do not preclude them from the desire to have a family, for example, kidney disease, rheumatoid arthritis, chronic lung disease, lupus, or heart disease. Often, though, the desire for a child is stronger than the woman's capacity for self-care, and self-care is crucial for women with chronic health conditions.

Women come into perinatal therapy with chronic illness possibly with a desire to have emotional support through their fertility journey. Often, they experience high levels of pregnancy-related fear and anxiety due to the risks of becoming pregnant and going through birth. Risk factors involved are preterm birth, low birth weight, impacts on the growth patterns in the fetus, or premature death and long-term illness of the mother (Gogoi & Unisa, 2017). High blood pressure and pre-eclampsia are also risk factors. Many women know of the risks and challenges they will face, which can exacerbate their fear of whether their condition and medication may impact their infant both in utero and post-birth whilst breastfeeding. Some women are also concerned about their ability to fulfil their responsibilities as a mother.

Many women may be having medical treatment throughout the pregnancy and birth, and this may place stress and anxiety on them and can increase deep-seated fears around health anxieties. Therapy offers the possibility to explore what the woman is deeply anxious about, which may not feel possible or plausible with their doctor or consultant. Going through pregnancy or getting close to birth, women can become unsure that this is the right decision for them and may go through intense ambivalence and can even doubt they want children. There are often fears that medication will stop working or that the change during pregnancy and postnatally may impact their medication and that the pain will be unbearable.

For the therapist, it is critical that there is no judgement or bias towards the woman's decisions around her fertility journey. However, there may be the need to juggle the woman's risk perceptions (often low, before pregnancy), which may change considerably if her chronic illness changes and her consultant is concerned for her own health and how it will be impacted by pregnancy and birth. As I said earlier, helping the woman juggle her desire for a child and the absolute need for self-care can be critical. Helping her to explore her fantasies and what reality may look like can also be helpful prior to her decision to embark on this journey.

Having a chronic illness and becoming a mum is difficult. Supporting a woman and sometimes her partner through such challenging circumstances can be rewarding yet complex and may feel like being on an emotional roller coaster at times. I would repeat my message: self-care for both client and therapist can be paramount.

Postpartum Psychosis

Postpartum psychosis can be particularly difficult to work with as a psychotherapist and may be impossible if the woman is experiencing active psychotic symptoms, due to a possible lack of available Adult. However, this doesn't preclude a mother from already being in psychotherapy and experiencing psychosis. I have worked with quite a few women with a diagnosis of postpartum psychosis. However, it is not easy, and requires a high level of input from a supervisor with experience in this type of client presentation.

Before taking on this type of client, I would need to confirm whether the psychosis is ongoing. If it is, there may not be enough capacity for the client to be present in the session. Even if the psychosis is not ongoing, capacity is essential, as clients who take strong antipsychotic medication may have little cognitive capacity at the level required for therapy to be useful and effective.

It is imperative that I know who the mother's support network is and to be in communication with the doctor, psychiatric team and any other mental health practitioners involved in her care. This is the case for any client with a mental health diagnosis, regardless of presentation, and particularly important for postpartum psychosis. Open communication and transparency between myself, my client and any other part of the psychiatric team is essential, so it is vital to open that communication. I believe it is incumbent on me to do this rather than the medical team. To be clear, the women I have worked with have mainly come to me post-discharge from inpatient psychiatric mother and baby units, by self-referral. Occasionally, women have come via suggestions from a medical clinician.

It is important to know that women can experience psychosis not only in the first few weeks post-birth but also some months after childbirth. I have had clients who were actively psychotic in their assessment session, five or even six months post-birth, and who needed to be immediately referred to psychiatric services. I always advocate this is done with the woman's knowledge and preferably with her in the room, so that any conversation around the referral is absolutely transparent. This is particularly important with psychosis, as high levels of paranoia are one of the symptoms.

Difficulties can come from a woman being referred by their partner. Partners are normally really good at spotting that something is wrong with the mother but may have no real concept of the severity of the situation. Many partners contact me first to ask for my help because they are concerned about their partner's behaviour or emotions. Ethically, I cannot see the mother unless she contacts me. Once in a while, I will be asked for couples therapy, often in the hope that I will see how unwell the mother is and perhaps 'do' something. Again, ethically, it is impossible to offer couples therapy if one partner is unwilling to participate and in the initial assessment session, I take time to explore the willingness of both mother and partner.

For those women who have come into psychotherapy post-discharge from an inpatient psychiatric mother and baby unit, the fear and trauma of their experience are the main foci of our attention, as is helping the mother to bond and attach to and interact with the infant, if this is needed. The mother is often still very unwell, usually with symptoms of extremely depressed mood, and often an inability to get out of bed. Usually, she is on strong anti-psychotic medication, which can mean that therapeutic engagement is challenging. Due to the symptoms of mania that are present in postpartum psychosis, a lack of sleep for many nights in a row is a good indication that something is seriously wrong. This may mean that she is prescribed medication that brings deep sleep, and it can take a while for the woman to come out of the groggy state this type of medication can bring the following morning. This means real thought and attention is needed on the timing of appointments.

I find it helpful to explore the symptoms of the psychosis, i.e. what she believed when she was in a psychotic state. This exploration can bring helpful information, as many women speak of their psychosis as centred around a fear of having their baby removed from them, by a partner or by 'someone'. This is such a common fear for many perinatal mothers, regardless of whether they are unwell or not. In England, not many infants are taken into care, and those that are usually have experienced deprivation, abuse or are from lone-parent households in which the parent is seriously struggling to care for the child (ONS, 2022b). Part of my role is to reassure the mother, and to give her some clarity about the reality of this happening, i.e. that it is extremely unlikely. The sense that the partner will take the child away is almost always catastrophic thinking too, although it is important to be sure this is only a fantasy. It is rare, but for some women, this may be a reality, and there may have been a threat made by the partner at some point.

Often, the woman has a high level of fear that she will become psychotic again. The experience of being psychotic and being taken into inpatient services is not necessarily at all pleasant, and can be perceived as highly traumatic. The thought of experiencing this again is often terrifying. This fear is often combined with the desire to go back to who she was before the psychosis (i.e. before the infant's birth). This desire adds a level of complexity to the work and it is important to gently explore how the mother feels about her infant. Many women with postpartum psychosis are absolutely bonded and attached to their infant. However, I would want to explore whether there is any sense that the infant is perceived as the cause of the psychosis.

The trauma from postpartum psychosis can be profound and is often combined with a powerful sense of shame. Many women seem utterly confused about why it happened and find it difficult to come to terms with. Some are fearful they may harm their baby, and some who are experiencing particularly dark thoughts may even speak of the baby and family members being better off without them. This might be when the partner is particularly well attached and bonded to the infant or if there is another caregiver, such as a nanny or childminder, to take care of the infant. Envy of those experiencing normal life can be intense and helping the mother to speak up about her disturbing thoughts can go a long way to dispelling them.

The work with postpartum psychosis is usually long term, and with each mother it takes a different amount of time to feel more positive. Using trauma techniques can be really helpful, although I am very hesitant about using EMDR with these clients, due to a concern that it might trigger psychosis. Using creative methods to help unlock the experience and to help the mother make meaning of her psychosis is useful. This type of work can be particularly challenging, and there is a good chance that the therapist may experience a strong parallel process, such as a sense of confusion, being dazed, in a trance, or even feeling manic, with pressure of speech in supervision, and when writing up notes.

For more information on working with this type of presentation, I have written a chapter about postpartum psychosis in my previous book on motherhood and mental illness (Haynes, 2022b). There is also a chapter on maternal trauma, which may offer more information on these two difficult presentations.

Maternal Trauma

Maternal trauma is not only birth trauma, it may be the trauma of infertility, miscarriage, termination for medical reasons (TFMR), stillbirth or neonatal death, rape and childhood sexual abuse. I encapsulate all of these with postpartum psychosis into what I term maternal trauma, which is any traumatic event from conception through to the postnatal period. It is also important to acknowledge that every person has a different capacity to cope with trauma. Some may develop post-traumatic stress disorder (PTSD), for others they may come through the traumatic event with no long-term symptoms.

For traumas experienced during conception and pregnancy, often the question I am most asked by women is "why?". This is often followed by a need for reassurance that it will not happen again. I am not an obstetrician, so I would never be able to answer such questions. In these instances, it is useful to direct the woman to charities that specialise in their particular type of trauma, as this may be a better way for them to gain answers. What is clear is that fear is a huge part of the therapy, as is coming to terms with not knowing or not being able to gain adequate answers about why. There is often a sense of failure as a woman, particularly with miscarriage, stillbirth or neonatal death, which can manifest in self-punishment, particularly for those women who are perfectionists, or who need to feel in control.

Grief forms a large part of the work and can take a considerable time to dissipate. There is also the difficulty of the woman's need for secrecy due to traumas such as rape, childhood sexual abuse, and TFMR and the shame that comes with them. For couples going through TFMR, they can face an almost impossible decision to make: whether to terminate their pregnancy, which may be at a later stage, or whether to carry the baby to term without knowing whether the baby will survive or not. In some countries, TFMR is not legally allowed, causing the mother to have to carry a baby to term that she may well know will die during birth or within the first few moments after birth or risking going to prison if she does terminate. This can take a terrible toll on the woman's mental and physical health and the 40 weeks of pregnancy can feel interminable.

Stillbirth and neonatal death happen to around 5000 babies per annum in the UK (SANDS, 2021). In the US, more than 21,000 babies were stillborn in 2021; that is around six in every 1,000 live births. Worldwide, around 5.1 million babies are stillborn or die in the neonatal period (Akuze et al., 2021).

Factors involved in the frequency of stillbirth are: ethnicity (Black women are more likely to experience it); age (women over 35 years of age); multiple births (i.e. women carrying triplets or quadruplets); low socioeconomic status (98% of stillbirth occurs in low or middle-income countries – Akuze et al., 2021); smoking; or a previous loss in pregnancy.

Becoming pregnant again can bring extreme levels of anxiety, which some women find almost impossible to control. Vocalising this anxiety can be very helpful, particularly if the woman is in fear of letting their midwife or obstetrician know about their anxiety. Women can feel a great deal of shame and may feel they are burdening their health care practitioners by constantly needing reassurance. Some women may be offered a home monitoring system to hear their baby's heartbeat. However, others I have worked with have said this can be counterproductive and even can increase their obsession and anxiety. Often, I have found that women simply need a holding environment once or twice a week to express their fears to me so that I can hear them and witness time passing with them. This may sound untherapeutic, yet if it alleviates some anxiety and allows the woman to know there is someone there to listen, this may be all she might need as reassurance to get her through the endless weeks of waiting.

The INTERSECT study (intersectstudy.org) shows that between 20 and 40% of mothers experience childbirth as traumatic, and around 4% go on to develop PTSD. Research by Beck, Watson and Gable (2018) showed that around 45% of women report experiencing birth as traumatic, and some practitioners consider birth trauma to be of international public health concern due to the high levels reported. Risk factors are prior mental health concerns and poor provision of perinatal services. The impact can be on maternal bonding, attachment and breastfeeding, and women can experience mental health concerns that can reoccur around the anniversary of the birth. Women who need surgery to repair damage post-birth can also experience discomfort or difficulties with sexual intimacy.

Some women experience PTSD due to intense fear that they or their baby were close to death during the traumatic birth. Cycles of rumination are common, and it can take a long time for women to come through their traumatic birth experience, meaning planning for future children may be put on hold or are put off permanently.

Treatment can focus on the trauma, disturbance, loss and grief, with sessions that are particularly painful. Space and time are needed for the depth of guilt, shame, grief and despair to materialise. Losing a yearned-for infant can be particularly difficult and painful because there is often no answer to the reason for the loss. The term 'unexplained' is often used by doctors or consultants around miscarriage, which is of little help to the couple involved. Many women talk of the madness of their grief and loss, and this can be disturbing for her partner and family, but also for the therapist too. Understanding enough about somatic symptoms, such as the pain women feel in their arms or breasts after the loss of their infant, can be helpful to normalise, as can the ongoing hormones that continue even after miscarriage or stillbirth and that can be deeply distressing to experience. Some women have said they are convinced they are still pregnant, even when they know they aren't, due to the hormones still in their system. This can feel utterly overwhelming, and the intense jealousy and rage towards those with a new, healthy baby can feel frightening. These feelings of jealousy and rage can come with feelings of intense shame and guilt, particularly if the woman needs to stay away from close friends or family who have given birth recently. It may also cause friction between close friends and relatives, which can be particularly painful and distressing if this tension causes an end to the friendship.

Historic Mental Health Difficulties

Also at play may be a woman's historic mental health difficulties. It is known that those who have experienced the severest of mental health conditions, such as bipolar disorder (Di Florio et al., 2013), or schizophrenia, are far more likely to experience a relapse during the perinatal period. It is also known that genetics contribute only a small part in risk and resilience in psychiatric disorders (Klengel, Dias & Ressler, 2016) and particularly for depressive disorders (Major Depressive Disorder Working Group of the Psychiatric GWAS Consortium – Power et al. 2017), although some genetic factors have been found for schizophrenia (Schizophrenia Working Group of the Psychiatric Genomics Consortium, 2014) and bipolar disorder (Muhleisen et al., 2014). This may be useful for some mothers to know, as many are concerned they will pass their mental illness onto their infant.

Considerations for women with historic mental illness may be around discontinuation of medication with pregnancy, as women who stop taking their psychotropic medication are far more likely to experience a relapse in their condition, particularly those who are taking mood stabilisers. For women who experience unplanned pregnancy, it is not safe for them to abruptly stop their medication. They will need help from their psychiatrist and will need to be referred for consultation so that ongoing medication and treatment can be discussed.

Our role for these women may again simply be a holding role. We cannot advise about medication and pregnancy. However, we can offer the space and time for a woman to explore how she is feeling and to voice any concerns she has. There may also be a need for the woman to learn to advocate for herself and her baby, being able to state what she needs and to help her ask for those needs to be met. She may also not know about the risks involved with her medication and breastfeeding.

It is helpful for therapists to have some knowledge about the risks of medication in pregnancy and when breastfeeding, as well as any concerns there may be about not taking medication. This would be mainly for information purposes, so the therapist knows what to look for in the client. In the UK, there is guidance published for psychotherapists and counsellors who have clients who want to withdraw from medication. The guidance helps to enable therapists to speak to clients regarding taking or withdrawing from prescribed medication, which is very helpful to access (Guy, Davies & Rizq, 2019). In the United States, the Substance Abuse and Mental Health Services Administration (SAMHSA) also issues guidance and training to mental health workers regarding the tapering of psychotropic medication. Many governments have guidelines like the UK and US. However, research by Read et al. (2023) showed that prescribers in many national health services are not properly informed about helping patients to taper their medication, in particular antidepressant medication. This is corroborated by Sørensen, Juhl Jørgensen and Munkholm (2022).

Self-Care

I would like to make self-care a primary objective when working in the perinatal field.

Self-care is advocated for a great deal in psychotherapy. We talk about self-care as supervisors and with our clients, but do we prioritise self-care for ourselves? Self-care is crucial in relational perinatal work because the therapist is a co-participant in the therapy: "the person of the clinician is the locus of successful psychotherapy" (Norcross & Guy, 2007, p. 3). Research shows that the therapist's well-being impacts treatment (Beutler, Machado & Neufeldt, 1994; Thériault et al., 2015) and expert psychotherapists recommend making self-care a primary objective for all mental health practitioners (Thériault et al., 2015).

Relational perinatal psychotherapy risks taking the therapist towards burnout because of the need to be in the process with the client. It asks more of the therapist than classical TA psychotherapy. I have experienced how close to burnout this work can take me, so I want to draw attention to burnout and the importance of self-care as a brake. It is so vital for therapists to recognise it in themselves, hopefully before their supervisor or therapist, and to do something to mitigate it.

Even before getting as far as being at risk of burnout, there can be a risk of the slow drip, drip, drip of something from the client (expectation, need, yearning, for example), which can permeate through the strongest of boundaries, particularly in times of stress. I can struggle when this slow drip from the client begins to feel overwhelming. What I may notice is that I don't look forward to seeing my client, or I may have a feeling that too much is required of me. It is at these times that I notice my defences rising, another clue that I need space to breathe and reconnect with myself.

Personally, when I am stressed, I go to a place of cognition, pressuring myself to be as good as possible. As a defence, it makes sense, but when working with a client, it means I may miss them as my defences are activated. This is where a solid understanding of my own drivers can be helpful, even if it does not necessarily stop the unconscious processes from occurring. I have found self-care to be crucial, and I know I must keep my self-care thoroughly integrated into my daily life. This means adequate time off, a broad client practice, knowing how many clients are too much and using my own therapy and supervision to explore my process with clients. No matter how long I have been practising, I need help to see and explore my own processes, so therapy and supervision are invaluable.

An example was during the pandemic when I needed help to keep my boundaries strong. It was all too easy to want to help the numerous clients who were struggling and reaching out for therapy. No matter our specialism, situations like the pandemic can bring out the rescuing and people-pleasing in many of us therapists. In particular, I found that perinatal clients were struggling so much more during this period, probably because many of them were home-schooling and trying to work at the same time, with children and partners all in the mix together. The levels of fear and anxiety were overly high in my clients and in their partners and children, if not at extreme levels. This was corroborated by research from many different countries (see Basu et al.'s 2021 study from 64 countries and Lebel et al., 2020, for further information). This meant I quickly found myself seeing many more clients than normal. This was fine for the short term, but with each subsequent lockdown, I noticed myself feeling more worn out. I could not initially escape anywhere on vacation either, one route for my self-care, which was also a problem. Luckily, once lockdown rules were relaxed, I could escape from work.

A part of self-care is the importance of having strong boundaries. Self-care and strong boundaries are both talked about within many different types of psychotherapy training. Still, my experience is that unless the trainee or therapist reaches a critical point of failure, such as multiple clients leaving, burnout, or even an ethical complaint against them, these two concepts remain talked about but are not truly integrated into practice despite the possible repercussions. I talked about the importance of strong boundaries in Chapter 4.

Conclusion

My aim in writing this chapter is to emphasise that work in perinatal psychotherapy can be disturbing, ethically charged, and may take a toll on the therapist. Although the work can be extremely fulfilling, it also has the possibility of being overwhelming and gruelling. It is not for everybody. I have highlighted some of the most complex of perinatal presentations. However, there are many more.

Self-care is so often spoken about, yet I doubt it is truly a part of many peoples' lives. Psychotherapists are naturally prone to being rescuers, and rescuers don't tend to place their own self above and beyond that of their clients. I want to emphasise how crucial it is to do so, and state that it is not ethical to place self-care at the bottom of the list. This is why I am a huge advocate for continuing therapy throughout our professional lives. It is all too easy to revert to script when stress and burnout begin to materialise, and this is precisely when it is important to have the support and help that is needed. This is exactly the same for mothers in their hour of need. If therapists are to be able to offer the care and help that is so needed in the perinatal period, they need to be able to model their own self-care.

13

INTERCONNECTIVITY THAT IS HUMAN BEING

The Inter-Relational

I want to end this book by offering a brief highlight of all the other influential and interconnected 'others' in an infant's development, all of which deserve their own TA theory. Like the mother, these influential others may also be pivotal to the infant. The roles of these influencing others are fundamentally interconnected with the development of the self and human being. I call the combination of all these influential others 'the inter-relational'. In this chapter, I want to offer an introduction to this inter-relationality. For me, each of these 'other' influences also offers much to be explored, and my hope is that inter-relationality could form part of the next stage in the development of this area of theory for TA.

Let's begin with some context. The development of the self in TA, through the focus on ego psychology, has its roots in Western philosophy, which is steeped in individualism. This means that individual achievement, the pursuit of new knowledge and scientific methods, independence, autonomy and the ability to be self-contained are often stroked as good. The focus is on the 'I' rather than the 'we'. This may mean that problem-solving, and even psychotherapy, may focus on individual, separate elements rather than seeing the problem through a holistic lens and recognising all the interconnections and inter-relationships that impact self-development. Emphasising the importance of these interconnections in human development shows that there can never be simply an 'I'; that this is, in fact, nonsense; there is always a 'we'. I also want to show the significance of the energy generated by this interconnectivity, this togetherness, the 'more than I', which I believe is physis. Introducing this interconnectivity for me is about acknowledging the 'we' in our human becoming and highlighting the 'we' as vitally important.

Some of the most profound difficulties people experience come from the interplay between themselves and pivotal, influencing others in their relationships. Humans do not become on their own, nor do they survive well in isolation. The Cambridge Dictionary states that inter-relationship is "the way in which two or more things or people are connected and affect one another" (2022), and this is why I have called this concept the inter-relational. I hope to briefly highlight the relational dynamics at play and

DOI: 10.4324/9781003365822-13

the influence each part can have on the development of the self. However, my aim is only to introduce inter-relationality. I believe that to develop the inter-relational in its entirety needs a group of transactional analysts, as it is complex. Apart from anything, I have found it difficult to show this concept diagrammatically, particularly when I know it needs to be seen in a moving, evolving, living, breathing way.

Within psychotherapy particularly, and indeed in our own TA literature, there is knowledge about the impact of abusive, traumatising and neglectful mothering. Yet, not enough is written about the other dynamic aspects of familial relationships, although McQuillin and Welford have written about family systems (2013). The inter-relational is more than family systems. It is not only the mother who plays a role within the familial system. I want to highlight the other parts in the inter-relational system that also have a signifi-cant role to play: fathers/partners, siblings, grandparents, significant others, the environment and the transgenerational. It is also essential to account for those people for whom 'family' may not necessarily mean the people they have a genetic connection to or have similarity with, such as those who are adopted. With the increasing use of artificial techniques for fertilisation, including sperm or egg donorship, those people who have been conceived in this way also need to be accounted for.

I am hyper-sensitive to the interconnection of the self and the family groups we are born into and the impact this continues to have on us during our lifetime. However, I now recognise that it is also possible to apply inter-relational theory to groups and organisations as well as the family. What I mean by this is that in all groups and organisations, there will be role players, just like there are in the inter-relational family unit. In organisations or in groups the maternal and paternal will be those who had the idea of the group or organisation in the first place. Siblings maybe those who are also impor-tant members of the group or organisation, such as directors. The transgen-erational aspects are also inherent within groups and organisations, as is the environment the group or organisation was born into and operates within. The diagrams below show the interconnectivity of humans and the environ-ment and the role the environment plays in shaping and impacting us in all aspects of these groups or organisations. Exploring these aspects is also possi-ble, highlighting the impact and influence the inter-relational has both inside and outside the family system.

The inter-relational is complicated. For instance, I can begin with the whole and break it down, or begin with the individual aspects and build it up. Because of my love of evolution, I have chosen to echo human develop-ment by building up the separate relational dynamics at play that are best represented in a two-dimensional (2D) format first. However, the approach may become more understandable if represented and thought about in three dimensions (3D), then adding in the fourth dimension of time, allowing for temporal elements – the continuing and evolving aspects of the before, the present and beyond. I will attempt to explain how the 3D elements add to and evolve the theory, later in the chapter.

The Nuclear Family

When I began thinking about interconnectivity, I called the nuclear family the 'intra-relationship' – meaning *within a single familial relationship*. Intra-relationship has been used before, as in Intra-Relational Accelerated Experiential Dynamic Psychotherapy (Lamagna & Gleiser, 2007). Lamagna also used it in describing 'self-relatedness' (2011). However, I find the term unhelpful, and confusing. It is also difficult to have two terms (intra-relational and inter-relational), one meaning the nuclear family and one encapsulating the multiple generations of the before, the present and beyond. Thus, I have incorporated them both into the term inter-relational.

To build context, I will start with the seven elements I describe in the nuclear family: the single-family system composed of mother, father, siblings, grandparents, self, significant others, and the environment. These are transitional elements and vulnerable to power, oppression and marginalisation. There is bi-directional and multidirectional movement between the elements. Each is affected by attachment and interconnection and will contain a multitude of its own elements and each has the ability to grow and change with time. There is also no order as to which element comes first, because, as with the chicken and egg scenario, what on earth does come first? I have chosen to show the elements intersecting in the area that is the shaded circle (in Figures 13.1, 13.2, 13.3 and 13.4), which is the 'self' and is initially a representation of the embryo/fetus or infant in Figure 13.1.

The Embryonic Stage

Although I represent the self in 2D format in Figure 13.1, I visualise it in 3D form, as a sphere, to represent the embryo. The external barrier or boundary of the embryo (the black line in Figure 13.1) is critical as protection and allows the fetus to form internally. The sphere represents 'the embryonic self'. The external boundary represents the container of safety and security; it is the skin, the boundary, and the container within which life can survive. Another 'container' that may be applied to this embryonic 'self' is the womb, which is also the safe container, providing the environment in which the fetus can grow and develop. If either of the boundaries of these two containers is breached, the embryo will die.

Outside the external boundary of the self is the environment. The environment in utero is crucially important to a fetus and can impact the gene presentation of the infant, which is known from scientific research and epigenetics. It is also known that events in early life (both in the womb and post-birth) are powerful in the way they can influence and impact susceptibility to certain

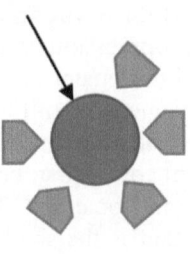

External boundary, e.g. skin

The impact and influence
of the Environment on the
development of the self is
shown by the shaded
arrows

Figure 13.1 The Embryonic Self

diseases throughout life (Gluckman et al., 2008) and gene presentation of the growing infant for the entirety of its life.

The environment, therefore, directly impacts the development of the self. The environment is so crucial to species survival that the scientific exploration of evolution now shows that the environment may directly impact the next generation through something called 'maternal effects', which I introduced in Chapters 1, 2 and 5.

Returning to the growth of the self, the baby stays within its safe container in the womb until the container is outgrown, and the birth of 'self' occurs, as the womb is no longer required. The infant is born into the world with its own safe container already formed, which is the skin. This metaphor of a safe container is useful and can be applied to many things. Other 'safe' containers might be the family unit, the earth's atmosphere and inanimate objects such as cars, planes, and boats, etc.

Mother and Father

The self comes into being with a 'mother' and a 'father', regardless of whether we know or have a relationship with them. Figure 13.2 shows the mother and father represented by two ovals, which are separate individuals yet meet and encircle the self.

I have used the terms 'mother' and 'father' because, at present, conception still requires an egg from 'mother' and sperm from 'father' to cause the fusion of gametes that brings forth a new individual or self. Conception is a great deal more complicated than this, and I hope that, by now, some of the complexities are more apparent.

The term 'father' would also encapsulate partner. Biologically, we see the 'father' in the traditional role of providing the sperm to fertilise the egg. Much like the maternal, the father/partner encapsulates so much more than simply the role of fertilisation. The father/partner is also not necessarily male.

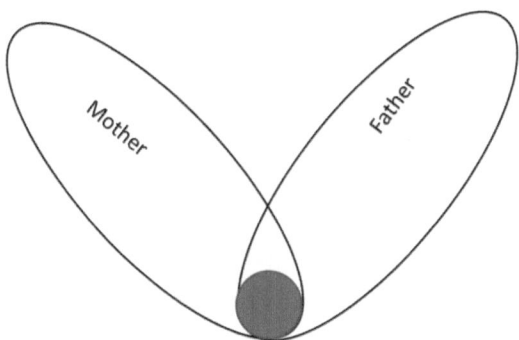

Figure 13.2 The Self with Representations of 'Mother' and 'Father' (2D)

However, it is essential not to get caught up in a biological argument regarding chromosomes, gender and sex, as there is no space here to explore biological implications.

The theory of the father/partner, in psychotherapy and psychoanalytic theory, recreates the patriarchal positioning of the father as a figurehead or authority figure to the infant. I find it more beneficial to highlight the father/partner as an inter-relational third, complementary and yet differentiated from the mother, with a very different but crucial role in the infant's life. This role is focused towards co-parenting and safety and security. If the mother's role is to be inwardly focused on the infant, and will include bonding, attachment, attunement and affect regulation, the role and identity the father/partner offers is one of support to the mother and also to focus the infant's gaze outwards towards the world around the infant.

What might this representation look like for a person who is adopted or is disconnected from either or both their birth parents, perhaps due to them being egg or sperm donors? This might be shown using a dotted line to form the 'mother' and/or the 'father' to represent the shadow of that person.

In Figure 13.3, the dotted line around 'mother' shows the shadow of a mother who passed away in childbirth yet who still influences the infant genetically and transgenerationally throughout the infant's lifetime, like a haunting. For example, this 'haunting' might materialise in the infant as prolonged grief, persistent yearning, and preoccupation with the shadow of the mother, impacting their ability to be emotionally available to those who are living. This type of haunting is likely to materialise in a multitude of different ways and may impact the infant physically, psychologically and emotionally. I have shown earlier in this book the severe consequences for the infant and family when the mother dies. In this representation (Figure 13.3), the father is still alive and part of the infant/self's world. For those who are adopted or

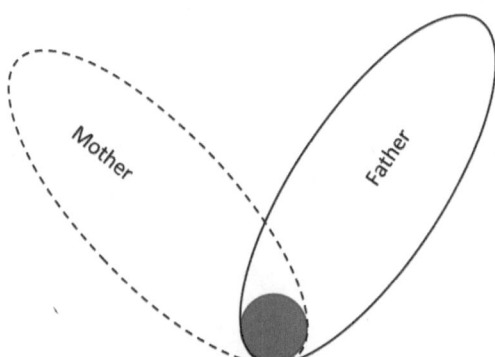

Figure 13.3 The Self with Representations of Father (alive), and Mother (who died in childbirth, shown by a dotted line) (2D)

who were perhaps conceived through donor egg and/or sperm we might also show both mother and father with a dotted line.

Others influence the nuclear family regardless of whether they are involved in the infant's life, such as the two sets of grandparents. For simplicity, I have combined the two sets into one. There may also be siblings, and/or step-siblings, too. Siblings are often significant factors in our lives. If there are no siblings, or siblings have been lost, either due to their death or separation through divorce, this loss or lack would again be represented through a dotted line. Significant others are represented because it would seem that many people have those who were influential at some point in their infancy, childhood, or later in life. Even when a child is neglected or seriously abused, they may speak of a neighbour, a teacher or possibly other friends or relatives who were part of their life and offered some form of recognition or care.

The final element, shown in Figure 13.4, is the environment, represented by the outer circle that encircles and encompasses all the other aspects. The word environment captures many meanings, such as the actual environment, ecology, culture, religion and spirituality. It may mean the womb, the family culture, or the atmosphere we live in, which provides the safety and ability to survive and provides all the nutrients and sustenance required, much like the womb. The environment encircles all the other elements and impacts each of them and is the safe container in which they function. As stated previously,

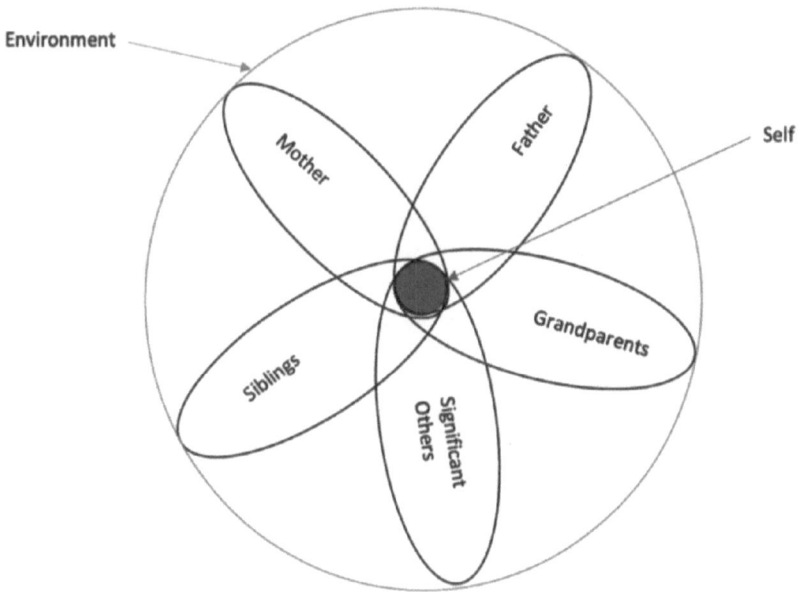

Figure 13.4 A 2D Representation of the Seven Interconnected Parts of the Nuclear Family

epigenetics shows that the environment in utero and within the first years of brain development post-birth and through into adulthood is a crucial influencing factor for psychiatric disorders and other diseases. Increasing evidence shows the impact of this on humans throughout their lives (see Ann Diamond Weinstein, 2016, for a comprehensive view).

The single nuclear family, including all its interconnecting component parts, interact as a team (or group) and help with the healthy development of the self. Each component or element has a role in developing the self. Each also has its own tolerance level it can work within. All interact together, and this interaction will also influence and impact the energy, growth, potential and physis of the self. I envisage them as depicted in the Venn diagram in Figure 13.4.

The quality of the elemental parts is important. If the mother, father, siblings, significant others and grandparents act and interact well together, and the environment offers good enough conditions, there will be growth, physis and resilience and the possibility of the 'self' reaching its potential. However, if one element is out of kilter or, perhaps, holds the self too tightly (through control or symbiotic relationship, for example), this may impact the energy in the self or sap it, causing the self to become stifled, suppressed or smothered. Equally, with a lack of guidance from the different elements and/or little interaction between the elements and the self, then the self may struggle, having undefined, unclear or even slack boundaries that are too sloppy and allow for too much movement in possibility for the self, wasting energy.

Pressure due to one element being out of kilter with the others, or perhaps outside their tolerance level, may mean that the development of the self could become lopsided. If one element is missing or is lacking, then development will still occur, yet growth might not be on a smooth trajectory. All the parts need to be in balance, as much as possible, and within their tolerances for the development of the self to be as healthy as possible. On top of this, the environment also impacts the energy and the expansion, growth and efficiency of the self. As the mother and father work together in partnership, if the tolerance level between these two partners is not right, or indeed there is friction between these and other elements, such as the grandparents, then this may also negatively impact the growth of the self.

The shape of each element in the diagrams above doesn't offer a real sense of the quantity and quality of their impact on the development of the self. Perhaps the mother might be seen as the most important structure for the infant and may be depicted with a much larger section, or with a stronger colour or line. Perhaps the father/partner would be more of a supporting structure, and if not present, or not present in the way needed, may be shown with a less intense outline or even a dotted line.

In Figure 13.4, the whole is much greater than the sum of the parts. For each 'self' to grow and develop in a healthy, functioning way, there is a need for these component or elemental roles to work together holistically. Each of the elements impacts energy. All are impactful. Finally, the environment for each and every 'self' will be different, just as it was different for the parents and grandparents who went before.

The Inter-Relational: A Dynamic Representation of Development

Suppose we now expand our thinking from a single nuclear family and bring in the intergenerational and temporal aspects of past, present and future and include them in the theory. In that case, I see this as the inter-relationality that is human becoming. Figure 13.5 shows how I envisage the 2D depiction of the component or elemental parts of the inter-relational. In this diagram, due to the expansion of each of the concepts, mother would become the maternal, father would become the paternal, grandparents and our ancestors would be included in the transgenerational. Significant others would not change, although significant others through the generations would be included. The category of siblings, however, may include aunts, uncles and cousins, to account for the siblings of each of the generations. The self also moves into alignment with all the other elements, as it is no longer about the development of the self only. This theory is more about the interconnectivity between these six human aspects within every one of us, and how they

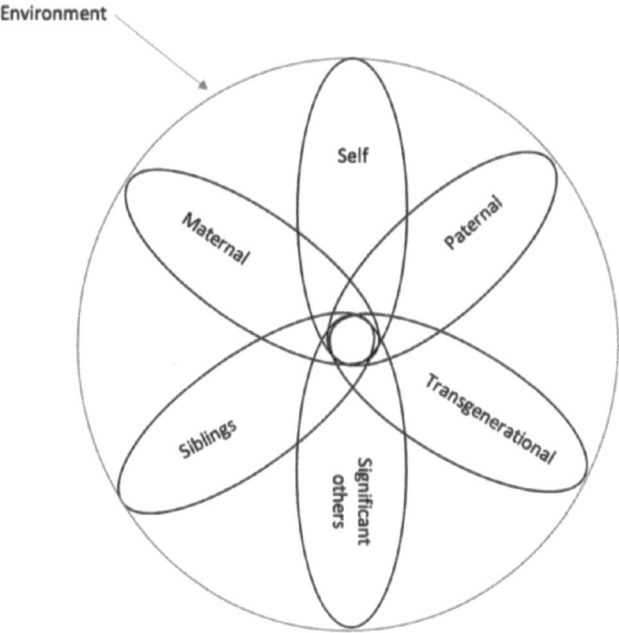

Figure 13.5 The 2D Depiction of the Inter-Relational

187

interact from the past, in the present, and into the future. All six are still held within the outer circle that is the environment.

Thinking in 2D has its limitations and does not account for and show inter-relationality as it truly is, which is as a dynamic system that is multigenerational and has no beginning and no end. It is infinite. In 3D form, there is an acknowledgement of the forward-moving growth force or physis.

Dependent upon how it is viewed, the 3D representation of the inter-relational, which would incorporate the generations that went before and those after, could perhaps be represented by a helix, a ceaseless spiral, a coil or even a spring, although it is difficult to represent it here on a two-dimensional page (see Figure 13.6). The direction of the spiral would be forwards and upwards and this forward movement would represent physis, the growth force. Each spiral revolution might, perhaps, be one generation, i.e. the nuclear family represented in Figure 13.4.

By viewing the inter-relational in a 3D form and viewing it like a spiral, it is easier to begin to think about what might happen if one of the elements is off-kilter, or unbalanced, or is over-influencing. For example, the spiral may not grow straight but may lean at an angle. Equally, if the spiral is represented tightly or loosely, then this might show the tightness or looseness of control within the intergenerations of that particular family. If one element holds too much control, the spiral will lose its shape and the energy and growth may be lopsided and off-centre.

Each one of the elements: maternal, paternal, transgenerational, siblings, significant others, the self, and the environment is a theory in its own right, and just as there is now some theory on the maternal, on Eco-TA and a great deal of theory on the self, theory for the other elements could be developed. This would hopefully capture all the many possibilities, elements and interactions within each one of the component parts.

As I said above, this may be for a group of transactional analysts to do, in order to combine a knowledge base broader than solely my own understanding of the maternal. Perhaps there are others in the TA community who might want to add to our theory and knowledge by writing about these other aspects.

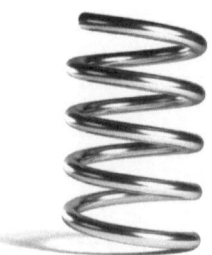

The direction of physis and growth

Figure 13.6 A 3D Representation of the Inter-Relational to Show the forward Movement of Physis and Growth

Conclusion

Giving space for the interconnectivity and inter-relationality in the development of human being is important. It is difficult to show and do it justice here in this chapter as I envisage it as much more than I have written. What I hope is clear is that a holistic lens is required when examining the development of human becoming, as it is never only about one element, the development of the self. It is about how we develop as human beings through our interconnections and inter-relations with the important others in our lives. I hope that by briefly introducing the inter-relational, I have acknowledged the 'we' in human development. No one develops on their own, or in a vacuum.

Connection, which I spoke about in the preface, is a vital and fundamental part of human being. Humans need self-connection and also connection to the environment. I see the emphasis around the world is on environmental concerns and this is right, it is vitally important for human survival. What I don't see being emphasised is the importance of human connection and particularly self-connection. Although I do see the negative aspects of a lack in connection – loneliness, isolation, mental illness and despair.

As Eco-TA highlights, everything in our world is interconnected. To evolve and grow transactional analytic theory, it would seem important to add 'interconnection' to the fundamental principles of TA.

14

A LIFETIME'S REDUCTION IN MENTAL ILLNESS?

Motherhood, and the maternal are transitional. From the moment of conceiving, women are constantly transitioning from one stage to another, and these transitions can be fraught with difficulty and disturbance. The maternal is about identity, vulnerability (control, choice and autonomy), difference, and particularly, loss and grief: the loss of the pre-pregnancy body, the loss of sense of self, the loss of time, space and energy, the loss of the pre-infant relationship between a couple. So many aspects of life before pregnancy are lost, let alone the loss and grief through miscarriage, termination for medical reasons, stillbirth, neonatal death and infertility. However, many elements of TA theory can be put to practical use to enable women through the disturbances and difficulties in these transitions. My aim in writing this book is to show how useful TA can be and how it can be applied to maternal disturbance. Another aim is to fill the gap in TA theory by including the maternal. I believe TA might benefit from incorporating the maternal into its psychotherapy training and into all the other fields, too, because it is such a fundamental aspect in the development of the self.

I am a strong advocate for TA relational psychotherapy for maternal disturbance and perinatal mental illness because it offers the possibility of long-lasting change for the mother. This change will positively impact her infant, her partner and her family. If this book encourages even a small percentage of TA practitioners to offer this type of treatment, it will have been worth writing it. At present, the only TA research we have for this treatment is my small-scale study, completed in 2019. If others are inspired, then I may fulfil a dream of a much larger longitudinal research study that would be wider in its scope and might even be worldwide. For the first time in many years, this now feels that it might be possible. This is exciting and could boost the profile of TA in the field of perinatal psychotherapy.

TA relational perinatal psychotherapy offers six vital benefits that help with the long-term reduction of maternal disturbance and mental illness. These six are:

1   Increasing the understanding of and capacity for relational connection in mothers, fathers and partners

                    DOI: 10.4324/9781003365822-14

2   A reduction in trauma, shame, stigma and silence – benefitting the long-term sense of self in the mother and boosting her self-connection

3   The possibility to change the attachment styles of both parents, but particularly the mother – benefitting parent–infant connection, bonding and regulatory processes

4   An increase in knowledge and understanding of, and possibility for behavioural change towards becoming the 'good enough' mother

5   Heightened attunement

6   Increasing the woman's ability and capacity for self-care – vital in long-term physical and psychological health.

Each of these six benefits also impacts the relationship between the mother and infant, the parent and infant, the couple's relationship, and is thus beneficial to the wider family and to society.

Within the chapters, my aim has been to show the nature and implications of silence within the maternal, and how relational psychotherapy can encourage women to speak out and be heard, particularly when experiencing difficulties in their perinatal journey. The silence might be due to guilt, shame and stigma, among other things. It might also be due to the mother's fear of speaking up and the risk of losing her infant. Psychotherapy offers an opportunity for women to overcome this very genuine fear, which hampers help-seeking behaviour due to fear of stigma and prejudice.

More than this, in writing this book, I am emphasising how crucial conception, pregnancy and the first 1,000 days of an infant's life are on the infant's ability to fulfil the huge potential and possibility they are born with, and this impacts all of us. The difference between someone's ability to thrive, rather than to simply survive, hinges on this fundamental foundational stage of life. Thus, supporting those who are essential caregivers at this hugely influential time seems vitally and absolutely necessary. Yet, as I have shown in each chapter, support for pregnancy, birth and parenting still remains neglected in many countries throughout the world and is neglected in TA theory and practice. Offering parents the possibility of psychological therapy as a form of treatment can go some considerable way to improving the parental journey.

I am also highlighting the fundamental importance of protocol, bringing this theory into the light rather than leaving it in the shadows where it has been for too long. Protocol is crucial, yet it remains largely unspoken about in TA and is certainly not researched or explored in the way it should be within the transactional analytic community. Among all the theories we have in TA, protocol is, for me, one of the most important theories of all. It is tied to human brain development and incorporates transgenerational protocol. Due to the encoding that occurs within protocol around safety and danger, and the relational patterns and attachment and regulatory processes, this may explain why it is impossible to change our protocol, and why it is the foundation stone in our potential, physis, and intuition. I believe protocol needs to be emphasised, expanded, researched and taught in a much greater way than at present. I have shown how protocol includes the fundamental interconnecting roles of attachment and affect regulation and how these are so important in human connection and interconnection, to self and to others, all of which are vital to remaining healthy and having a physical, mental, psychological, emotional and social state of well-being.

The birth of a child is filled with such possibility and potential. Yet, the transition to motherhood can be such a complex, personal, significant, disturbing and often difficult time for many women. This transition is no longer necessarily about choice because those who want to be mothers and those who can be are changing due to changes in fertility. Change may be around how many children to have, and it may also be due to more women delaying motherhood. In many parts of the world, parents no longer need large families due to the declining infant mortality rate. Wider access to contraception continues to be a high priority for the WHO, and in 2022, the global prevalence of contraceptive usage was up at 65% (WHO, 2023). Some parents are also actively choosing to have smaller families and for many couples, the choice may be to have no children. Change is also occurring in parenting due to the acceptability of single-sex parents in many countries, although in some, like Italy, for example, there has been a sudden, worrying and very recent reversal towards unacceptability, limiting adoption, surrogacy and the legal rights of same-sex couples.

Regardless of the changing nature of parenthood, impending motherhood is steeped with fantasy, yearning, and idealisation, and a desire to recreate the family of origin or, in contrast, to create the loving, stable family that wasn't available. As I said in the preface, this is often in contrast to the experience a woman has in becoming pregnant, being pregnant, giving birth and mothering. It is also the time in life with the most capacity to stir up historic relational difficulties and disturbing processes from infancy and childhood, and there is potential for undigested disturbances to be passed transgenerationally from mother to infant, as it has been in some families for many generations.

The transition to motherhood is a time of high expectations. These might include the assumption that falling pregnant will be easy; it might be a vision of having an uncomplicated, smooth pregnancy and for the birth process to also be smooth and relatively straightforward; there could be an expectation that the infant will fit into the life of the parents, rather than the parents having to refocus their lives to the needs of the child; and for the milestone stages to be met by the infant, or preferably for the infant to be considered 'forward' for their age, as a way to reinforce the parent's feelings of being the 'best' parents; finally, there is often an expectation that children will be reasonably happy and healthy and will mature into happy healthy adults, ready to repeat the process with their own children. Some of these expectations cannot or won't be met. If they are not, then this can disrupt and disturb the fantasies and longings inherent in motherhood.

Due to multi-factorial and often highly complex reasons, some women are more likely to find the transition to motherhood difficult. If this transition is a struggle, there is often a ripple effect on the entire family and on society. Yet, it is the negative impact on the child that is of most concern. It is imperative that TA psychotherapists offer treatment so that more women know that help is there when and if they need it. The more help offered, the more supported women and parents will feel, benefitting them and their infants.

Still today, in 2023, women globally do not have the choice and control they wish for over their bodies through reproduction, pregnancy and birth. Many women continue to remain vulnerable and dependent on their partners, on the medical profession, and on others to help with the care for their children post-birth. The battle with patriarchy continues, as does the battle for parity of pay and legal rights. The battle to improve women's experiences of pregnancy, birth and motherhood also continues. From the moment of conception, women are vulnerable to criticism, pain of judgement, and negative exposure. It is uncanny that, as soon as she is known to be pregnant, a woman can become objectified at a societal level.

Dr Simone Holligan, a lecturer at the University of Guelph states

> Western society tends to view the female body as an object that should be constantly inspected and evaluated, and valued for its utility and ability to give pleasure ... Societal pressures to maintain the ideal female body may be heightened during pregnancy.
>
> (2023)

There has been a recent rise in media coverage, and photos of naked and heavily pregnant influential women in social media and within magazines. This began with Demi Moore in 1991, followed by Britney Spears, Eva Herzigova, Jessica Simpson, Christina Aguilera, Mariah Carey, Nia Long, Monica Belluci, Cindy Crawford and Claudia Schiffer, to name just a few. These models and film stars have impacted both the sexualisation and the beauty ideal of pregnancy in the media, with a rise in self-objectification in pregnancy (Beech et al., 2020). This has added to the pressure of being the perfect mother, as women feel they now also need to have the perfect body, as quickly as possible, post-birth. The concerns cited by pregnant and post-birth women are as follows: concerns around body shape and size, with concurrent body shaming and a rise in body dysmorphia; breastfeeding and fear of not being able to breastfeed, as well as the impact this will have on the body; disordered eating post birth due to fear of body shape; and a rise in body dissatisfaction (Brock et al., 2021). Objectification still occurs in pregnancy, as women continue to report being questioned by all manner of people about all sorts of intimate things to do with their fetus and birth. This simply wouldn't occur outside pregnancy. Strangers still seem to think it is acceptable to enter a woman's personal space and place their hand on her bump, for example, as if it was publicly acceptable. How can we help to curb this sexualisation and objectification of mothers?

This book has focused on maternal disturbance and mental illness yet has also touched on the difficulties and challenges fathers, partners, adoptive and foster parents can experience. This book can only ever touch on a small proportion of the aspects of motherhood and disturbance in the maternal. It has been designed to open up dialogue around what maternal mental illness really is – illness or systemic failure due to lack of care and support for parents. What I hope the book does highlight is how relational transactional analysis psychotherapy can offer successful and useful treatment for the myriad of different presentations. I believe it also shows that TA psychotherapy can offer both a practical and useful alternative to medication or that it can be offered alongside medication.

The book has taken a relational treatment approach focused towards TA practitioners and has offered my thoughts and experience about relational perinatal psychotherapy: what it is, why it is so fundamental, the importance of the role of 'mother' in attachment and affect regulation, and the differences I perceive when working in the perinatal space as opposed to working with other mental illnesses. I have explored common TA concepts such as protocol, assessment, diagnosis, treatment planning, groups, and couples work. I have also included chapters on: creativity, as a powerful way of unlocking silence and stuckness; fathers and partners, and how they can also feel disturbed through this transitional period; complex presentations, disturbance and the importance of self-care for psychotherapists working in this field; and finally, I have situated the maternal within what I call the inter-relational, showing how the maternal is only one part of the interconnectivity that is human becoming. Throughout the book, where possible, I have integrated new conventions on neuroscience and neurobiology with therapeutic interventions. The book is grounded in research and my own clinical experience.

I hope I have shown how effective working with groups can be. For many years, I felt that group work might be contra-indicated with maternal clients, as I found women did not want to share their experiences in a group scenario. This would appear to be true for women who are at a very low ebb, or who are experiencing high levels of anxiety. The idea of speaking in a group space would seem to amplify any low mood or anxiety, which is not helpful. However, it is quite apparent that if the group is about a specific area of the parenting journey, then this is more attractive. In particular, groups around loss, miscarriage or the fertility journey seem to be well attended, and this would include groups focused towards partners too. As with many groups, sharing an experience within the group space can be so helpful as a way of feeling less alone and isolated, particularly if what is offered is an opportunity for reflection and exploration. Also, for fertility groups, having members who are at different stages of their fertility journey can be reassuring to those who are at an earlier stage.

My goal with treatment is always to hope that the mother or parent in front of me can gain enough understanding and curiosity in themselves that they continue to develop and grow emotionally and psychologically and I hope that I can offer something towards them experiencing a lifetime reduction in their mental illness. I do acknowledge, however, that sometimes this is not possible.

Thank you for reading this book. I hope it will stimulate conversation and dialogue about all aspects of the family, not only the maternal, and encourage other practitioners to work in and research this area. My own pathway is to continue to explore, research, add to and evolve TA theory, but not on my own. So far, and for too many years, my work has felt incredibly lonely and isolating, with a lack of understanding about and discounting of what is such a crucial part of the development of the self, with few other clinicians interested in it, or acknowledging how important mothers and parents are. Perhaps this will now change.

REFERENCES

Addis, M.E., & Mahalik, J.R. (2003). Men, masculinity, and the contexts of help seeking. *American Psychologist*, *58*, 5–14. https://doi.org/10.1037/0003-066x.58.1.5

Adewuya, A.O., & Afolabi, O.T. (2005). The course of anxiety and depressive symptoms in Nigerian postpartum women. *Archives of Women's Mental* Health, *8*(4), 257–259.

Admon, L.K., Winkelman, T.N.A., Moniz, M.H., Davis, M.M., Heisler, M., & Dalton, V. (2017). Disparities in chronic conditions among women hospitalized for delivery in the United States, 2005–2014. *Obstetrics & Gynecology*, *130*(6), 1319–1326. https://doi.org/10.1097/AOG.0000000000002357

Akuze, J., Cousens, S., Lawn, J.E., Waiswa, P., Godeev, V.S., Arnold, F., Croft, T., Baschieri, A., & Blencowe, H. (2021). Four decades of measuring stillbirths and neonatal deaths in Demographic and Health Surveys: Historical review. *Population Metrics*, *19*(Suppl. 1), 8. https://doi.org/10.1186/s12963-020-00225-0

Al-Allaf, A.W., Dunbar, K.L., Sallum, N.S., Nosratzadeh, B., Templeton, K.D., & Pullar, T. (2002). A case-control study examining the role of physical trauma in the onset of fibromyalgia syndrome. *Rheumatology*, *41*(4), 450–453. https://doi.org/10.1093/rheumatology/41.4.450

Aldridge, B., & Stilman, R. (2024). Unmasking neurodiversity: Revisiting the relationship between core self and sense of self to examine common neurodivergent script decisions. *Transactional Analysis Journal*, *54*(1), 47–62. https://doi.org/10.1080/03621537.2024.2286576

Allen, J.R. (2003). Concepts, competencies, and interpretive communities. *Transactional Analysis Journal*, *33*, 146–147.

Allotey, J., Stallings, E., Monet, M., Yao, M., Chatterjee, S., Kew, T., Debenham, L., Llavall, A.C., Dixit, A., Zhou, D., Balaji, R., Lee, S., Qiu, X., Yuan, M., Coomar, D., van Wely, M., van Leeuwen, E., Kostova, E., & Kunst, H. (2020). Clinical manifestations, risk factors and maternal and perinatal outcomes of coronavirus disease 2019 in pregnancy: Living systematic review and meta-analysis. *British Medical Journal*, *370*, m3320. https://doi.org/10.1136/bmj.m3320

American Psychological Association (APA) (2009). The changing role of the modern day father. www.apa.org/pi/families/resources/changing-father#:~:text=Today%27s%20father%20is%20no%20longer,facing%20physical%20or%20psychological%20challenges

American Psychological Association (APA) (2013). *Diagnostic and Statistical Manual of Mental Disorders, Fifth Edition.* Arlington, VA: American Psychiatric Association.

American Psychological Association, Boys and Men Guidelines Group. (2018). *APA guidelines for psychological practice with boys and men.* www.apa.org/about/policy/psychological-practice-boys-men-guidelines.pdf

Anchesi, S.D., Corallo, F., DiCara, M., Quartarone, A., Catalioto, R., Cucinotta, F., & Cardile, D. (2023). Autism and ADHD: A literature review regarding their impacts on parental divorce. *Children (Basel)*, *10*(3), 438. https://doi.org/10.3390/children10030438

Andreasen, N. (2011). A journey into chaos: Creativity and the unconscious. *Mens Sana Monographs*, *9*(1), 42–53. https://doi.org/10.4103/0973-1229.77424

Anokye, R., Acheampong, E., Budu-Ainooson, A., Obeng, E.I., & Akwasi, A.G. (2018). Prevalence of postpartum depression and interventions utilized for its management. *Annals of General Psychiatry*, *17*, 1–8. https://doi.org/10.1186/s12991-018-0188-0

Apprey, M. (2019). "Scripting" inhabitations of unwelcome guests, hosts, and ghosts: Unpacking elements that constitute transgenerational haunting. *Transactional Analysis Journal*, *49*(4), 339–351. https://doi.org/10.1080/03621537.2019.1650234

Arcaya, M.C., Arcaya, A.L., & Subramanian, S.V. (2015). Inequalities in health: Definitions, concepts and theories. *Global Health Action*, *8*(1), 27106. https://doi.org/10.3402/gha.v8.27106

Aristotle. (1994). Aristotle's "De anima" (Z. ben I. ben Shealtiel Hen, Trans., G. Bos, Ed.). Leiden: Brill. (Original work published 429 BC)

Atuhaire, C., Brennaman, L., Cumber, S.N., Rukundo, G.Z., & Nambozi, G. (2020). The magnitude of postpartum depression among mothers in Africa: A literature review. *Pan African Medical Journal*, *37*(89). https://doi.org/10.11604/pamj.2020.37.89.23572

Austin, M.P., Frilingos, M., Lumley, J. Hadzi-Pavlovic, D., Roncolato, W., Acland, S., & Parker, G. (2008). Brief antenatal cognitive behaviour therapy group intervention for the prevention of postnatal depression and anxiety: A randomised controlled trial. *Journal of Affective Disorders*, *105*(1), 35–44. https://doi.org/10.1016/j.jad.2007.04.001

Australian Institute of Health and Welfare (2021). *Maternal deaths*. AIHW, Australian Government. www.aihw.gov.au/getmedia/8b25ea27-7304-441c-b708-48c65ce5bb55/Maternal-deaths.pdf.aspx?inline=true 26.04.2023

Aydin, E., Glasgow, K.A., Weiss, S.M., Khan, Z., Austin, T., Johnson, M.H., Barlow, J., & Lloyd-Fox, S. (2022). Giving birth in a pandemic: Women's birth experiences in England during COVID-19. *BMC Pregnancy and Childbirth*, *22*, 304. https://dpo.prg/10.1186/s12884-022-04637-8

Ayoub, K., Shaheen, A., & Hajat, S. (2020). Postpartum depression in the Arab region: A systematic literature review. *Clinical Practice & Epidemiology in Mental Health*, *16*(Suppl-1), 142–155. https://doi.org/10.2174/1745017902016010142

Ayyub, H., Sarfraz, M., Mir, K., & Sala, F. (2018). Association of antenatal depression and household food insecurity among pregnant women: A cross-sectional study from slums of Lahore. *Journal of Ayub Medical College Abbottabad*, *30*(3), 366–371.

Baggaley, R.F., Ganaba, R., Filippi, V., Kere, M., Marshall, T., Sombié, I., et al. (2007). Detecting depression after pregnancy: The validity of the K10 and K6 in Burkina Faso. *Tropical Medicine and Interntional Health*, *12*(10), 1225–1229.

Ball Cooper, E., Anderson, J.L., Sharp, C., Langley, H.A., & Venta, A. (2021). Attachment, mentalization, and criterion B of the alternative *DSM-5* model for personality disorders (AMPD). *Borderline Personality Disorder and Emotional Dysregulation*, *8*(23). https://doi.org/10.1186/s40479-021-00163-9

Barragan-Jason, G., Loreau, M., de Mazancourt, C., Singer, M.C., & Parmesan, C. (2023). Psychological and physical connections with nature improve both human well-being and nature conservation: A systematic review of meta-analyses. *Biological Conservation*, *277*, e109842. https://doi.org/10.1016/j.biocon.2022.109842

Barrett, J. (2022). Fertility preservation for transgender individuals. *Reproduction and Fertility, 3*(2), C11–C13. https://doi.org/10.1530/RAF-21-0090

Barrett, L., Fraser, L., Noyes, J., Taylor, J., & Hackett, J. (2023). Understanding parent experiences of end-of-life care for children: A systematic review and qualitative evidence synthesis. *Palliative Medicine, 37*(2), 178–202. https://doi.org/10.1177/02692163221144084

Basu, A., Kim, H.H., Basaldua, R., Choi, K.W., Charron, L., Kelsall, N., Hernandez-Diaz, S., Wyszynski, E.F., & Koenen, K.C. (2021). A cross-national study of factors associated with women's perinatal mental health and wellbeing during the COVID-19 pandemic. *PloS ONE, 16*(4), e0249780. https://doi.org/10.1371/journal.pone.0249780

Battle, C., Salisbury, A.L., Schofield, C.A., & Ortiz-Hernandez, S. (2013). Perinatal antidepressant use: Understanding women's preferences and concerns. *Journal of Psychiatric Practice, 19*(6), 443–453. https://doi.org/10.1097/01.pra.0000438183.74359.46

Bauer, A., Parsonage, M., Knapp, M., Iemmi, V., Adelaja, B. (2014). The costs of perinatal mental health problems. *LSE & Centre for Mental Health*. http://eprints.lse.ac.uk/59885/1/__lse.ac.uk_storage_LIBRARY_Secondary_libfile_shared_repository_Content_Bauer%2C%20M_Bauer_Costs_perinatal_%20mental_2014_Bauer_Costs_perinatal_mental_2014_author.pdf

Bauer, A., Knapp, M., Parsonage, M. (2016). Lifetime costs of perinatal anxiety and depression. *Journal of Affective Disorders, 1*(192), 83–90. https://doi.org/10.1016/j.jad.2015.12.005

Bauer, A., Knapp, M., Matijasevich, A., Osório, A., & Silvestre de Paula, C. (2022a). The lifetime costs of perinatal depression and anxiety in Brazil. *Journal of Affective Disorders, 319*, 361–369. https://doi.org/10.1016/j.jad.2022.09.102

Bauer, A., Garman, E., Besada, D., Field, S., Knapp, M., & Honikman, S. (2022b) Costs of common perinatal mental health problems in South Africa. *Global Mental Health, 9*, 429–438. https://doi.org/10.1017/gmh.2022.48

Beck, C.T., Watson, S., & Gable, R.K. (2018). Traumatic childbirth and its aftermath: Is there anything positive? *The Journal of Perinatal Education, 27*(3), 175–184. https://doi.org/10.1891/1058-1243.27.3.175

Beebe, B., Jaffe, J., Markese, S., Buck, K., Chen, H., Cohen, P., Bahrick, L., Andres, H., & Feldstein, S. (2010). The origins of 12-month attachment: A microanalysis of 4-month mother–infant interaction. *Attachment & Human Development, 12*(1–2), 3–141. https://doi.org/10.1080/14616730903338985

Beebe, B., Lachmann, F., Markese, S., & Bahrick, L. (2012). On the origins of disorganized attachment and internal working models: Paper I. A dyadic systems approach. *Psychoanalytic Dialogues, 22*(2), 253–272. https://doi.org/10.1080/10481885.2012.666147

Beech, O.D., Kaufmann, L., & Anderson, J. (2020). A systematic literature review exploring objectification and motherhood. *Psychology of Women Quarterly, 44*(4), 521–538. https://doi.org/10.1177/0361684320949810

Beeghly, M. (1997). Emergence of symbolic play: Perspectives from typical and atypical development. In J. Burack, R. Hodapp, & E. Zigler (Eds.), *Handbook of mental retardation and development* (pp. 240–289). New York: Cambridge University Press.

Behrman, R.E., & Butler, A.S. (2007). *Preterm birth: Causes, consequences, and prevention*. Committee on Understanding Premature Birth and Assuring Healthy Outcomes. National Academy of Sciences. www.nap.edu/catalog/11622

Benoit, D. (2004). Infant–parent attachment: Definition, types, antecedents, measurement and outcome. *Paediatrics and Child Health, 9*(8), 541–545. https://doi.org/10.1093/pch/9.8.541

Bergström M. (2013). Depressive symptoms in new first-time fathers: Associations with age, sociodemographic characteristics, and antenatal psychological well-being. *Birth, 40*, 32–38.

Berne, E. (1949). The nature of intuition. *Psychiatric Quarterly, 23*(2), 203–226. https://doi:.org/10.1007/BF01563116

Berne E. (1957). Ego states in psychotherapy. *The American Journal of Psychotherapy, 11*, 293–309.

Berne, E. (1961). *Transactional analysis in psychotherapy*. New York: Grove Press.

Berne, E. (1966/1994). *Principles of group treatment*. Menlo Park, CA: Shea Books. Republished in 1994.

Berne, E. (1970). *Sex in human loving*. New York: Simon & Schuster.

Berne, E. (1975[1972]). *What do you say after you say hello?: The psychology of human destiny*. New York: Grove Press.

Berne, E. (1976[1962]). Classification of positions, *Transactional Analysis Bulletin, 1*(3), 23.

Berne, E. (1977a). Primal images and primal judgments. In E. Berne, *Intuition and ego states* (pp. 67–97). San Francisco, CA: TA Press. (Original work entitled "Intuition IV: Primal images and primal judgment," published 1955).

Berne, E. (1977b). The nature of intuition. In E. Berne, *Intuition and ego states: The origins of transactional analysis* (P. McCormick, Ed.) (pp. 1–31). Pleasanton, CA: TA Press. (Original work published 1949)

Best, M., & Neuhauser, D. (2004). Ignaz Semmelweis and the birth of infection control. *BMJ Quality & Safety, 13*, 233–234. https://dx.doi.org/10.1136/qshc.2004.010918

Beutler, L.E., Machado, P.P.P., & Neufeldt, S.A. (1994). Therapist variables. In A.E. Bergin & S.L. Garfield (Eds.), *Handbook of psychotherapy and behavior change* (4th ed., pp. 229–269). New York: John Wiley & Sons.

Billert, H. (2007). Tokophobia – a multidisciplinary problem. *Ginekologia Polska, 78*(10), 807–811. PMID: 18200974.

Bion, W. (1962). *Learning from experience*. London: Karnac.

Bion, W.R. (1967). *Second thoughts*. London: Heinemann (Maresfield reprints).

Bird, G., & Cook, R. (2013). Mixed emotions: The contribution of alexithymia to the emotional symptoms of autism. *Translational Psychiatry, 3*(7), e285. https://doi.org/10.1038/tp.2013.61

Bollas, C. (1987). *The shadow of the object: Psychoanalysis of the unthought known*. New York: Columbia University Press.

Bollas, C. (2021). *Three characters: Narcissist, borderline, manic depressive*. Bicester, Oxon: Phoenix Publishing House.

Boots Family Trust Alliance, Netmums, Institute of Health Visiting, Tommy's, The Royal College of Midwives. (2013). *Perinatal mental health experiences of women and health professionals*. London: Boots Family Trust

Bowlby, J. (1982). Attachment and loss: Retrospect and prospect. *American Journal of Orthopsychiatry, 52*(4), 664–678. https://doi.org/10.1111/j.1939-0025.1982.tb01456.x

Brandthe, B., & Kvande, E. (2016). Masculinity and fathering alone during parental leave. *Men and Masculinities, 21*(1). https://doi.org/10.1177/1097184X16652659

Bretherton, I. (1992). The origins of attachment theory: John Bowlby and Mary Ainsworth. *Developmental Psychology, 28*(5), 759–775. https://doi.org/10.1037/0012-1649.28.5.759

Broadwell, M.M. (20 February 1969). Teaching for learning (XVI). https://edbatista.typepad.com/files/teaching-for-learning-martin-broadwell-1969-conscious-competence-model.pdf

Brock, R.L., Ramsdell, E.L., Sáez, G., & Gervais, S.J. (2021). Perceived humanization by intimate partners during pregnancy is associated with fewer depressive symptoms, less body dissatisfaction, and greater sexual satisfaction through reduced self-objectification. *Sex Roles, 84*, 285–298. https://doi.org/10.1007/s11199-020-01166-6

Bronte-Tinkew, J., Moore, K. A., Matthews, G., & Carrano, J. (2007). Symptoms of major depression in a sample of fathers of infants: Sociodemographic correlates and links to father involvement. *Journal of Family Issues, 28*(1), 61–99. https://doi.org/10.1177/0192513X06293609

Bruner, J. (1990). *Acts of meaning*. Cambridge, MA: Harvard University Press.

Bureau of Labor Statistics, United States Department of Labor (2023). *Employment Characteristics of Families – 2022*. USDL-23-0723. www.bls.gov/news.release/pdf/famee.pdf

Burman, J.T., Green, C.D., & Shanker, S. (2015). On the meanings of self-regulation: Digital humanities in service of conceptual clarity, *Child Development, 86*(5), 1507–1521. https://doi.org/10.1111/cdev.12395

Caizzi, C. (2012). Embodied trauma: Using the subsymbolic mode to access and change script protocol in traumatized adults. *Transactional Analysis Journal, 42*(3), 165–175. https://doi.org/10.1177/036215371204200302

Cambridge English Dictionary (2022). Cambridge, UK: Cambridge University Press.

Cameron, E.E., Sedov, I.D., & Tomfohr-Madsen, L.M. (2016). Prevalence of paternal depression in pregnancy and the postpartum: An updated meta-analysis. *Journal of Affective Disorders, 206*, 189–203. Https://doi.org/10.1016/j.jad.2016.07.044

Campbell, A.M. (2020). An increasing risk of family violence during the COVID-19 pandemic: Strengthening community collaborations to save lives. *Forensic Science International Reports, 2*, 100089. https://doi.org/10.1016/j.fsir.2020.100089

Carey, N. (2012). *The epigenetics revolution: How modern biology is rewriting our understanding of generics, disease and inheritance*. London: Icon Books.

Carlson, D.L., Petts, R., & Pepin, J. (2020). US couples' divisions of housework and childcare during COVID-19 pandemic. *SocArXiv*. https://doi.org/10.31235/osf.io/jy8fn

Carson, D.K., & Becker, K.W. (2004). When lightning strikes: Reexamining creativity in psychotherapy. *Journal of Counseling & Development, 82*, 111–115.

Cavarero, A. (1990/1995). *In spite of Plato: Feminist rewriting of ancient philosophy* (Trans. S. Anderlini-D'Onofrio and Á. O'Healy). Cambridge, UK: Polity Press.

Centre on the Developing Child (n.d.). Harvard University – Key Concepts https://developingchild.harvard.edu/science/key-concepts/

Centre on the Developing Child (n.d.). *Resilience* (InBrief). www.developingchild.harvard.edu; www.youtube.com/shorts/HdmTvGxfrRo

Centre on the Developing Child (2013). *The science of neglect* (InBrief). www.developingchild.harvard.edu; www.youtube.com/watch?v=bF3j5UVCSCA

Centers for Disease Control and Prevention (CDC) (2020). *Vital signs, identifying maternal depression – Missed opportunities to support moms*. www.cdc.gov/reproductivehealth/vital-signs/identifying-maternal-depression/VS-May-2020-Maternal-Depression_h.pdf

Centers for Disease Control and Prevention (CDC) (2022). *Working together to reduce black maternal mortality*. www.cdc.gov/healthequity/features/maternal-mortality/index.html

Centre for Mental Health and London School of Economics (2014). *The costs of perinatal mental health problems*. www.lse.ac.uk?LSEHealthAndSocialCare/aboutUs/PSSRU/home.aspx

Chhabra, J., Li, W., & McDermott, B. (2022). Predictive factors for depression and anxiety in men during the perinatal period: A mixed methods study. *American Journal of Men's Health, 16*(1). https://doi.org/10.1177/15579883221079489

Chesley, N. (2011). Stay-at-home fathers and breadwinning mothers: Gender, couple dynamics, and social change. *Gender & Society*, *25*(5), 642–664. https://doi.org/10.1177/0891243211417433

Chiesa, C. (2012a). Scripts in the sand: Sandplay in transactional analysis psychotherapy with children. *Transactional Analysis Journal*, *42*(4), 285–293. https://doi.org/10.1177/036215371204200407

Chiesa, C. (2012b). Sognare il sogno: Il gioco della sabis [Dreaming the dream: The sandplay]. In Itaca Association (Eds), *Incontrare il bambino giocando* [Meeting the child while playing] (pp. 179–191). Bergamo: Edizioni Junior.

Chiesa, C. (2014). On the seashore of an endless world, children play. *Transactional Analysis Journal*, *44*(2), 128–141. https://doi.org/10.1177/0362153714539916

Chin, K., Wendt, A., Bennett, I.M., & Bhat, A. (2022). Suicide and maternal mortality. *Current Psychiatry Reports*, *24*(4), 239–275. https://doi.org/10.1007/s11920-022-01334-3

Choy, A. (1990). The winner's triangle. *Transactional Analysis Journal*, *20*(1). https://doi.org/10.1177/036215379002000105

Chung, H. (2021). *Shared care, father's involvement in care and family well-being outcomes: A literature review*. Government Equalities Office. https://assets.publishing.service.gov.uk/media/6017fd418fa8f53fc739255d/Shared_care_and_well-being_outcomes-_Literature_review.pdf

Chung, H., Seo, H., Forbes, S., & Birkett, H. (2020). *Working from home during the COVID-19 lockdown: Changing preferences and the future of work*. Report for the project Work Autonomy, Flexibility and Work–Life Balance. Canterbury, UK: https://research.birmingham.ac.uk/en/publications/working-from-home-during-the-covid-19-lockdown-changing-preferenc

Chzhen, Y., Gromada, A., & Rees, G. (2019). *Are the world's richest countries family friendly? Policy in the OECD and EU*. Florence: UNICEF Office of Research.

Clark, B.D. (1991). Empathic transactions in the deconfusion of child ego states. *Transactional Analysis Journal*, *21*(2), 92–98. https://doi.org/10.1177/036215379102100204

Cleghorn, E. (2021). *Unwell women: A journey through medicine and myth in a man-made world*. London: Weidenfeld & Nicolson.

Cochran, S., & Rabinowitz, F. (2003). Gender-sensitive recommendations for assessment and treatment of depression in men. *Profession Psychology: Research and Practice*, *34*(2), 132–140. https://doi.org/10.1037/0735-7028.34.2.132

Condon, J.T., Boyce, O., & Corkindale, C.J. (2004). The first-time fathers study: A prospective study of the mental health and wellbeing of men during the transition to parenthood. *Australian & New Zealand Journal of Psychiatry*, *38*, 56–64. https://doi.org/10.1111/j.1440-1614.2004.01298x

Cooke, L. (2022). *Bitch: What does it mean to be female*. London: Transworld Publishers.

Coontz, S. (2005). *Marriage, a history: From obedience to intimacy or how love conquered marriage*. New York: Viking.

Cornell, W.F. (2008a). "My body is unhappy": Somatic foundations of script and script protocol. In W.F. Cornell (Ed.), *The Meech Lake papers*. Pleasanton, CA: TA Press.

Cornell, W.F. (2008b). *Explorations in transactional analysis: The Meech Lake papers*. Pleasanton, CA: TA Press.

Cornell, W.F. (2010). Aspiration or adaptation?: An unresolved tension in Eric Berne's basic beliefs. *Transactional Analysis Journal*, *40*(3–4), 243–253. https://doi.org/10.1177/036215371004000309

Cornell, W.F. (2011). SAMBA, TANGO, PUNK: Commentary on paper by Steven H. Knoblauch. *Psychoanalytic Dialogues*, *21*(4), 428–436. https://doi.org/10.1080/10481885.2011.595323

Cornell, W.F. (2015). Play at your own risk: Games, play and intimacy. *Transactional Analysis Journal, 44*(4), https://doi.org/10.1177/0362153714559921

Cornell, W.F. (2019). *At the interface of transactional analysis, psychoanalysis and body psychotherapy*. London, New York: Routledge.

Cornell, W.F., & Bonds-White, F. (2001) Therapeutic relatedness in transactional analysis: The truth of love or the love of truth. *Transactional Analysis Journal, 31*, 71–93. https://doi.org/10.1177/036215370103100108

Cornell, W.F., & Landaiche, N.M. III. (2005). Impasse e intimita nella coppia terapeutica o di counselling: l'influenza del protocollo [Impasse and intimacy in the therapeutic or consultative couple: The influence of protocol]. *Rivista Italiana di Analisi Transazionale e Metodologie Psicoterapeutiche, 11*, 35–60.

Cornell, W.F., & Landaiche, N.M. III. (2006). Impasse and intimacy: Applying Berne's concept of script protocol. *Transactional Analysis Journal, 36*(3), 196–213. https://doi org/10.1177/03621537060300304

Cornell, W.F., & Landaiche, N.M. III (2008). Nonconscious processes and self-development: Key concepts from Eric Berne and Christopher Bollas. In W.F. Cornell (Ed.), *The Meech Lake papers*. Pleasanton, CA: TA Press.

Coulson, J. (2022). *Opinion-editorial: Reflecting on progress in maternal health in China*. UNFPA opinion piece originally published on CGTN website on 9 October 2022. https://news.cgtn.com/news/2022-10-09/Reflecting-on-progress-in-maternal-health-in-China–1dZ5CCiRVCM/index.html

Cowles-Boyd, L. & Boyd, H.S. (1980a). Play as a time structure. *Transactional Analysis Journal, 10*, 5–7.

Cowles-Boyd, L. & Boyd, H.S. (1980b). Playing with games: The game/play shift. *Transactional Analysis Journal, 10*, 8–11.

Coxon, K., Turienzo, C.F., Kweekel, L., Goodarzi, B., Brigante, L., Simon, A., & Lanau, M.M. (2020). The impact of the coronavirus (COVID-19) pandemic on maternity care in Europe. *Midwifery, 88*, 102779. https://doi.org/10.1016/j.midw.2020.102779

Craig, L., & Churchill, B. (2020). Dual-earner parent couples' work and care during COVID-19. *Gender, Work & Organization.online first*. https://doi.org/10.1111/gwao.12497

Cropley, A.J. (2011). Definitions of creativity. In M.A. Runco & S.R. Pritzker (Eds), *Encyclopedia of creativity* (pp. 511–524). Cambridge, MA: Academic Press.

Csíkszentmihályi, M. (1990). *Flow: The psychology of optimal experience*. New York: Harper & Row.

Csíkszentmihályi, M. (1996). *Creativity: Flow and the psychology of discovery and invention*. New York: Harper Collins.

Csíkszentmihályi, M., & Csíkszentmihályi, I.S. (Eds.). (1988). *Optimal experience: Psychological studies of flow in consciousness*. New York: Cambridge University Press.

Dadi, A.F., Akalue, T.Y., Baraki, A.G., & Wolde, H.F. (2020). Epidemiology of postnatal depression and its associated factors in Africa: A systematic review and meta-analysis. *PLoS One, 15*(4), e0231940. https://doi.org/10.1371/journal.pone.0231940

Damon, W., & Hart, D. (1982). The development of self-understanding form infancy through adolescence. *Child Development, 53*(4), 841–864. https://doi.org/10.2307/1129122

Daniels, E., Arden-Close, E., & Mayers, A. (2020). Be quiet and man up: A qualitative questionnaire study into fathers who witnessed their partner's birth trauma. *BMC Pregnancy and Childbirth, 20*, 236. https://doi.org/10.1186/s12884-020-02902-2

Darwin, Z., Domoney, J., Iles, J., Bristow, F., Siew, J., & Sethna, V. (2021). Assessing the mental health of fathers, other co-parents, and partners in the perinatal period:

Mixed methods evidence synthesis. *Frontiers in Psychiatry*, *11*, 585479, 1–18. https://doi.org/10.3389/fpsyt.2020.585479

Darwin, Z., Galdas, P., Hinchliff, S., Littlewood, E., McMillan, D., McGowan, L., & Gilnody, S. on behalf of the Born and Bred in Yorkshire (BaBY) team. (2017). Fathers' views and experiences of their own mental health during pregnancy and the first postnatal year: a qualitative interview study of men participating in the UK Born and Bred in Yorkshire (BaBY) cohort. *BMC Pregnancy and Childbirth*, *17*(45). https://doi.org/10.1186/s12884-017-1229-4

Dawson, P., Auvray, B., Hay-Smith, J. Jaye, C., & Gauld, R. (2022). Social determinants and inequitable maternal and perinatal outcomes in Aotearoa New Zealand. *Women's Health*, *18*. https://doi.org/10.1177/17455065221075913

Dennis, C.L., Falah-Hassani, K., & Shiri, R. (2017). Prevalence of antenatal and postnatal anxiety: Systematic review and meta-analysis. *British Journal of Psychiatry*, *210*(5), 315–323. https://doi.org/10.1192/bjp.bp.116.187179

De Sutter, P., Kira, K., Verschoor, A., & Hotimsky, A. (2002). The desire to have children and the preservation of fertility in transsexual women: A survey. *International Journal of Transgenderism*, *6*(3), 3–97.

Dethier, D., & Abernathy, A. (2020). Maintaining certainty in the most uncertain of times. *Birth*, *47*(3), 257–258. https://doi.org/10.1111/birt.12496

Dharani, K. (2015). *The biology of thought: A neuronal mechanism in the generation of thought – a new molecular model*. eBook ISBN: 9780128011614. https://doi.org/10.1016/B978-0-12-800900-0.00003-8

Di Florio, A., Forty, L., Gordon-Smith, K., Heron, J., Jones, L., Craddock, N., & Jones, I. (2013). Perinatal episodes across the mood disorder spectrum. *JAMA Psychiatry*, *70*, 168–175. https://doi.org/10.1001/jamapsychiatry.2013.279

DiPietro, J.A., Costigan, K.A., Voegtline, K.M. (2015). Studies in fetal behavior: Revisited, renewed, and reimagined. *Monographs of the Society for Research in Child Development*, *80*(3), vii, 1–94. https://doi.org/10.1111/mono.v80.3. PMID: 26303396; PMCID: PMC4835043.

Duarte, J., Martinez, C., & Tomicic, A. (2020). Episodes of meeting in psychotherapy: An empirical exploration of patients' experiences of subjective change during their psychotherapy process. *Research in Psychotherapy*, *23*(1), 440. https://doi.org/10.4081/ripppo.2020.440

Edelstein, R.S., Chopik, W.J., Saxbe, D.E., Wardecker, B.M., Moors, A.C., & LaBelle, O.P. (2017). Prospective and dyadic associations between expectant parents' prenatal hormone changes and postpartum parenting outcomes. *Developmental Psychobiology*, *59*(1), 77–90. https://doi.org/10.1002/dev.21469

Edelstein, R.S., Wardecker, B.M., Chopick, W.J., Moors, A.C., Shipman, E.L., & Lin, N.J. (2015). Prenatal hormones in first-time expectant parents: Longitudinal changes and within-couple correlations. *American Journal of Human Biology*, *27*(3), 317–325. https://doi.org/10.1002/ajhb.22670

Edoka, I.P., Petrou, S., & Ramchandani, P.G., (2011). Healthcare costs of paternal depression in the postnatal period. *Journal of Affective Disorders*, *133*, 356–360. https://doi.org/10.1016/j.jad.2011.04.005

Eggermont, K., Beeckman D., Van Hecke, A., Delbaere, I., & Verhaeghe, S. (2017). Needs of fathers during labour and childbirth: A cross-sectional study. *Women and Birth*, *30*(4), 188–197. https://doi.org/10.1016/j.wombi.2016.12.001

English, F. (1972). Rackets and Real Feelings: Part II. *Transactional Analysis Bulletin*, *2*(1), 23–25. https://doi.org/10.1177/036215377200200108

Eri, T.S., Blix, E., Downe, S., Vedeler, C., & Nilsen, A.B.V. (2022). Giving birth and becoming a parent during the COVID-19 pandemic: A qualitative analysis of 806 women's responses to three open-ended questions in an online survey. *Midwifery*, *109*, Article 103321. https://doi.org/10.1016/j.midw.2022.103321

REFERENCES

Eriksson, C., Salander, P., & Hamberg, K. (2007). Men's experiences of intense fear related to childbirth investigated in a Swedish qualitative study. *Midwifery*, *4*(4), 409–418. https://doi.org.10.1016/j.midw.2005.10.002

Eriksson, C., Westman, G., & Hamberg, K. (2005). Experiential factors associated with childbirth-related fear in Swedish women and men: A population-based study. *Journal of Psychosomatic Obstetrics & Gynecology*, *26*(1), 63–72. https://doi.org/10.1080/01674820400023275

Erskine, R.G. (Ed.). (2010a). *Life scripts: A transactional analysis of unconscious relational patterns*. London: Karnac.

Erskine, R.G. (Ed.) (2010b). *Life scripts: Definitions and points of view*. www.integrativetherapy.com/en/articles.php?id=76

Etheridge, J., & Slade, P.P. (2017). "Nothing's actually happened to *me*": The experiences of fathers who found childbirth traumatic. *BMC Pregnancy & Childbirth*, *17*(1), 1–15. https://doi.org/10.1186/s12884-017-1259-y

Ettenber, M., Bieleninik, L., Epstein, S., & Elefant, C. (2021). Defining attachment and bonding: overlaps, differences and implications for music therapy clinical practice and research in neonatal intensive care units. *International Journal of Environmental Research and Public Health*, *18*(4), 1733. https://doi.org/10.3390/ijerph18041733

Ettinger, B.L. (2006). *The matrixial borderspace*. Minneapolis, MN: University of Minnesota Press.

Ettinger, B.L. (2010). (M)Other re-spect: Maternal subjectivity, the ready-made mother-monster and the ethics of respecting, *Studies in the Maternal*, *2*(1). www.mamsie.bbk.ac.uk/back_issues/issue_three/mother_respect.html

European Commission (2022). *Eurostat: Archive: Statistics on employment characteristics of households*. Revision as of 11.00, 1 June 2022. https://ec.europa.eu/eurostat/statistics-explained/index.php?title=Statistics_on_employment_characteristics_of_households&oldid=568074#Overview_of_employment_in_EU_households

European Union Priorities for 2019–24. https://europa.eu/european-union/about-eu/priorities_en

Fawcett, E.J., Fairbrother, N., Cox, M.L., White, I.R., & Fawcett, J.M. (2019). The prevalence of anxiety disorders during pregnancy and the postpartum period: A multivariate Bayesian meta-analysis. *Journal of Clinical Psychiatry*, *80*(4), 18r12527. https://doi.org/10.4088/JCP.18r12527

Figueiredo, B., Canário, C., Tendais, I., Pinto, T.M., Kenny, D.A., & Field, T. (2018). Couples' relationship affects mothers' and fathers' anxiety and depression trajectories over the transition to parenthood. *Journal of Affective Disorders*, *238*, 204–212. https://doi.org/10.1016/j.jad.2018.05.064

Firestein, M.R., Dumitriu, D., Marsh, R., & Monk, C. (2022). Maternal mental health and infant development during the COVID-10 pandemic. *JAMA Psychiatry*, *79*(10), 1040–1045. https://doi.10.1001/jamapsychiatry.2022.2591

Fitzgerald, M. (2020). *Blaming the mother*. http://professormichaelfitzgerald.eu/wp-content/uploads/Blaming-the-Mother-Article-by-Prof.-Michael-Fitzgerald-Opinion-GP-Ireland.pdf

Flouri, E., & Buchanan, A. (2003). The role of father involvement in children's later mental health. *Journal of Adolescence*, *26*(1), 63–78. https://doi.org/10.1016/S0140-1971(02)00116-1

Fonagy, P., Steele, M., Steele, H., Moran, G.S., & Higgitt, A.C. (1991). The capacity for understanding mental states: the reflective self in parent and child and its significance for security of attachment. *Infant Mental Health Journal*, *12*(3), 201–218. https://doi.org/10.1002/1097-0355(199123)12:3<201::AID-IMHJ2280120307>3.0.CO;2-7

Fonagy, P., Gergely, G., Jurist, L.E., & Target, M. (2004). *Affect regulation, mentalization, and the development of the self*. London: Karnac.

Friedman, S. (2018). How Our Careers Affect Our Children. *Harvard Business Review*, November 14th, 2018. https://hbr.org/2018/11/how-our-careers-affect-our-children

Friedman, R.S., & Förster, J. (2010). Implicit affective cues and attentional tuning: An integrative review. *Psychological Bulletin, 136*(5), 875–893. https://doi.org/10.1037/a0020495

Fromm-Reichman, F. (1948). Notes on the development of treatment of schizophrenics by psychoanalytic psychotherapy. *Psychiatry, 11*(3), 263–273.

Furness, P.J., Vogt, K., Ashe, S., Taylor, S., Haywood-Small, S., & Lawson, K. (2018). What causes fibromyalgia? An online survey of patient perspectives. *Health Psychology Open*. https://doi.org/10.1177/2055102918802683

Gallagher, J. (2020). Fertility rate: "Jaw-dropping" global crash in children being born. BBC News, Health 15 July 2020. www.bbc.co.uk/news/health-53409521

Galton, F. (1875). The history of twins, as a criterion of the relative powers of nature and nurture. *Journal of the Royal Anthropological Institute, 5*, 391–406 (Reprinted in *International Journal of Epidemiology*, 2012, *41*, 905–911.

Galvez-Sánchez, C.M., Duscheck, S., & Reyes Del Paso, G.A. (2019). Psychological impact of fibromyalgia: Current perspectives. *Psychology Research and Behavior Management, 12*, 117–127. https://doi.org/10.2147/PRBM.S178240

Gayol, G.N. (2004). Codependence: A transgenerational script. *Transactional Analysis Journal, 34*(4), 312–322. https://doi.org/10.1177/036215370403400404

George, C., Lalitha, A.R.N., Anotony, A., Kumar, A.V., & Jacobs, K.S. (2016). Antenatal depression in coastal South India: Prevalence and risk factors in the community. *International Journal of Social Psychiatry, 62*(2), 141–147. https://doi.org/10.1177/0020764015607919

Gergely, G., & Watson, J.S. (1996). The social biofeedback theory of parental affect-mirroring: The development of emotional self-awareness and self-control in infancy. *International Journal of Psychoanalysis, 77*(6), 1181–1212.

Gettler, L.T., McDade, T.W., Feranil, A.B., & Kuzawa, C.W. (2011). Longitudinal evidence that fatherhood decreases testosterone in human males. *Proceedings of the National Academy of Sciences, 108*(39), 16194–16199. https://doi.org/10.1073/pnas.1105403108

Gluckman, P.D., Hanson, M.A., Cooper, C., & Thornburg, K.L. (2008). Effect of in utero and early-life conditions on adult health and disease. *The New England Journal of Medicine, 359*(1), 61–73. https://doi.org/10.1056/NEJMra0708473

Gogoi, M., & Unnisa, S. (2017). Chronic Diseases during Pregnancy and Birth Outcome: A Study Based on Tertiary Hospital of Mumbai. *Women and Health, 3*(2), 61–69. https://doi.org/10.17140/WHOJ-3-123

Goulding, R., & Goulding, M. (1976). Injunctions, Decisions, and Redecisions. *Transactional Analysis Journal, 6*(1), 41–48. https://doi.org/10.1177/036215377600600110

Greenberg, L.S., & Goldman, R.N. (2008). *Emotion-focused couples therapy: The dynamics of emotion, love, and power*. Washington, DC: American Psychological Association

Greer, J. Lazenbatt, A., & Dunne, L. (2014). "Fear of childbirth" and ways of coping for pregnant women and their partners during the birthing process: A salutogenic analysis. *Evidence Based Midwifery, 12*, 95–100.

Guy, A., Davies J., & Rizq, R. (Eds) (2019). *Guidance for psychological therapists: Enabling conversations with clients taking or withdrawing from prescribed psychiatric drugs*. London: APPG for Prescribed Drug Dependence.

Hantsoo, L., Podcasy, J., Sammel, M., Epperson, C.N., & Kim, D.R. (2017). Pregnancy and the acceptability of computer-based versus traditional mental health treatments. *Journal of Women's Health (Larchmt)*, 26(10), 1106–1113. https://doi.org/10.1089/jwh.2016.6255

Hargaden, H. (2016). The role of the imagination in an analysis of unconscious relatedness. *Transactional Analysis Journal*, *46*(4), 311–321. https://doi.org/10.1177/0362153716662624

Hargaden, H., & Schwartz, J. (2007). Editorial. *European Journal of Psychotherapy and Counselling*, *9*(1).

Haynes, E. (2019). *"Hear Us Speak": Listening to women's experiences of perinatal distress and the Transactional Analysis psychotherapy treatment they received*. PhD thesis. http://usir.salford.ac.uk.id/eprint/51465/?template=banner

Haynes, E. (2022a). Bridging the gap between research and practice: Using creative methods to research. *Transactional Analysis Psychotherapy*, *52*(2), 134–147. https://doi.org/10.1080/03621537.2022.2019406

Haynes, E. (2022b). *Motherhood and mental illness: A relational treatment approach.* London and New York: Routledge.

Haynes, E. (2023). The maternal: An integral part of Eco-TA. *Transactional Analysis Journal*, *53*(1), 67–79. https://doi.org/10.1080/03621537.2023.2152549

Hildingsson, I., Johansson, M., Fenwick, J., Haines, H., & Rubertsson, C. (2014). Childbirth fear in expectant fathers: Findings from a regional Swedish cohort study. *Midwifery*, 30(2), 242–247. https://doi.org/10.1016/j.midw.2013.01.001

Hofberb, K., & Brockington, I. (2000). Tokophobia: An unreasoning dread of childbirth. A series of 26 cases. *British Journal of Psychiatry*, *176*, 83–85. https://doi.org/10.1192/bjp.176.1.83

Hoffman, K., Trawalter, S., Axt, J.R., & Oliver, M.N. (2016) Racial bias in pain assessment and treatment recommendations, and false beliefs about biological differences between blacks and whites. *The Proceedings of the National Academy of Sciences (PNAS)*, *113*(16), 4296–4301. https://doi.org/10.1073/pnas.1516047113

Holligan, S. (2023). *Commentary: Why we need to accept the pregnant body as a valued form*. News University of Guelph. https://news.uoguelph.ca/2023/03/why-we-need-to-accept-the-pregnant-body-as-a-valued-form/

Holtby, M.E. (1979). Interlocking Racket Systems. *Transactional Analysis Journal*, 9(2), 131–135. https://doi.org/10.1177/036215377790090218

Howard, L.M., Khalifeh, H. (2020). Perinatal mental health: A review of progress and challenges. *World Psychiatry*, *19*(3), 313–327. https://doi.org/10.1002/wps.20769

Hoyert, D.L. (2020). *Maternal mortality rates in the United States, 2020*. NCHS Health E-Stats. 2022. https://dx.doi.org/10.15620/cdc:113967

Hung, K.J., Tomlinson, M., le Roux, I.M., Dewing, S., Chopra, M., & Tsai, A.C. (2014). Community-based prenatal screening for postpartum depression in a South African township. *International Journal of Gynaecology and Obstetrics*, *126*(1), 74–77. https://doi.org/10.1016/j.ijgo.2014.01.011

Iles, J., Slade, O., & Spiby, H. (2011). Posttraumatic stress symptoms and postpartum depression in couples after childbirth: The role of partner support and attachment. *Journal of Anxiety Disorder*, *25*(4), 520–530. https://doi.org/10.1016/j.janxdis.2010.12.006

Insan, N., Weke, A., Rankin, J., & Forrest, S. (2022). Perceptions and attitudes around perinatal mental health in Bangladesh, India and Pakistan: A systematic review of qualitative data. *BMC Pregnancy and Childbirth*, *22*(293). https://doi.org/10.1186/s12884-022-04642-x

Institute for Research on Poverty. (2020). *Involved fathers play an important role in children's lives*. www.irp.wisc.edu/resource/involved-fathers-play-an-important-role-in-childrens-lives/#_edn7

Jantzen, G. (2004). *Foundations of violence*. London: Routledge.

Jia, R., Ayling, K., Chalder, T., Massey, A., Broadbent, E., Coupland, C., & Vedhara, K. (2020). Mental health in the UK during the Covid-19 pandemic: Cross-sectional analyses from a community cohort study. *BMJ Open, 10*, e040620. https://doi.10.1136/bmjopen-2020-040620

Johanson, R., Newburn, M., & Macfarlane, A. (2002). Has the medicalisation of childbirth gone too far? *British Medical Journal, 324*(7342), 892–895. https://doi.org/10.1136/bmj.324.7342.892

Jones, I., Chandra, P.S., Dazzan, P., & Howard, L.M. (2014). Bipolar disorder, affective psychosis, and schizophrenia in pregnancy and the post-partum period. *Lancet, 384*(9956), 1789–1799. https://doi.org/10.1016/S0140-6736(14)61278-2

Jones, W.H.S. (1923). *Hippocrates*, translated by W.H.S. Jones. London: William Heinemann; New York: G.P. Putnam's Sons.

Kahler, T. (1975). Drivers: The Key to the Process of Scripts. *Transactional Analysis Bulletin, 5*(3), 280–284. https://doi.org/10.1177/036215377500500318

Kahn, W.A. (1990). Psychological conditions of personal engagement and disengagement at work. *Academy of Management Journal, 33*(4), 692–724. https://doi.org/10.2307/256287

Kanner, L. (1949). Problems of nosology and psychodynamics of early infantile autism. *The American Journal of Orthopsychiatry, 19*, 416–426.

Karpman, S. (1968). Fairy tales and script drama analysis. *Transactional Analysis Bulletin, 7*(26), 39–43

Keleman, S., & Adler, S. (2000). Couples therapy as a formative process. *Journal of Couples Therapy, 10*(2), 49–59.

Kennell, J.H., & Klaus, M.H. (1984). Mother–infant bonding: Weighing the evidence. *Developmental Review, 4*(3), 275–282. https://doi.org/10.1016/S0273-2297(84)80008-8

Kersten, I., Lange, A.E., Haas, J.P., Fusch, C., Lode, H., Hoffman, W., & Thyrian, J.R. (2014). Chronic diseases in pregnant women: Prevalence and birth outcomes based on the SNiP-study. *BMC Pregnancy and Childbirth, 75*. https://doi.org/10.1186/1471-2393-14-75

Khalifa, D.S., Glavin, K., Bjertness, E., & Lien, L. (2015). Postnatal depression among Sudanese women: Prevalence and validation of the Edinburgh Postnatal Depression Scale at 3 months postpartum. *International Journal of Women's Health, 7*, 677–684. https://doi.org/10.2147/IJWH.S81401

Klaus, M.H., & Kennell, J.H. (1970). Mothers separated from their newborn infants. *Pediatric Clinics of North America, 17*(4), 1015–1037. https://doi.org/10.1016/s0031-3955(16)32493-2

Klengel, T., Dias, B.G., & Ressler, K.J. (2016). Models of intergenerational and transgenerational transmission of risk for psychopathology in mice. *Neuropsychopharmacology, 41*(1), 219–231. https://doi.org/10.1038/npp.2015.249. Epub 18 August 2015.

Knight, M., Bunch, K., Tuffnell, D., Shakespeare, J., Kotnis, R., Kenyon, S., & Kurinczuk, J.J. (Eds.) on behalf of MBRRACE-UK (2019). *Saving lives, improving mothers' care: Lessons learned to inform maternity care from the UK and Ireland Confidential Enquiries into Maternal Deaths and Morbidity 2015–17*. Oxford: National Perinatal Epidemiology Unit, University of Oxford.

Knudson Martin, C., & Mahoney, A.R. (2009). *Couples, gender and power: Creating change in intimate relationship*. New York: Springer Publishing.

Koch, B.D., & Jones, B.L. (2018). Supporting parent caregivers of children with life-limiting illness. *Children (Basel), 5*(7), 85. https://doi.org/10.3390/children5070085

Kohut, H. (1971). *The analysis of the self: A systematic approach to the psychoanalytic treatment of narcissistic personality disorders*. Chicago, IL: University of Chicago Press.

Konkel, L. (2018). The brain before birth: Using fMRI to explore the secrets of fetal neurodevelopment. *Environmental Health Perspectives*, *126*(11). https://doi.org/10.1289/EHP2268

Kottler, J.A., & Hecker, L.L. (2002). Creativity in therapy: Being struck by lightning and guided by thunderstorms. *Journal of Clinical Activities, Assignments & Handouts in Psychotherapy Practice*, *2*(2), 5–21. https://doi.org/10.1300/J182v02n02_02

Kraemer, G.W. (1992). A psychobiological theory of attachment. *Behavioral Brain Science*, *15*(3), 493–511. https://doi.org/10.1017/S0140525X00069752

Kristen-Antonow, S., Sodian, B., Perst, H., & Licata, M. (2015). A longitudinal study of the emerging self from 9 months to the age of 4 years. *Frontiers of Psychology*, *10*(6), 789. https://doi.org/10.3389/fpsyg.2015.00789

Kwan, B., Dimidjian, S., & Rizvi, S. (2010). Treatment preference, engagement and clinical improvement in pharmacotherapy versus psychotherapy for depression. *Behaviour Research and Therapy*, *48*(8), 799–804. https://doi.org/10.1016/j.brat.2010.04.003

Ladge, J.J., Humberd, B.K., Baskerville Watkins, M., & Harrington, B. (2015). Updating the organization MAN: An examination of involved fathering in the workplace. *Academy of Management Perspectives*, *29*(1), 152–171. https://www.jstor.org/stable/43822079

Lamagna, J. (2011). Of the self, by the self, and for the self: An intra-relational perspective on intra-psychic attunement and psychological change. *Journal of Psychotherapy Integration*, *21*(3), 280–307. https://doi.org/10.1037/a0025493

Lamagna, J., & Gleiser, K.A. (2007). Building a secure internal attachment: An intra-relational approach to ego strengthening and emotional processing with chronically traumatized clients. *Journal of Trauma & Dissociation*, *8*(1), 25–52. https://doi.org/10.1300/J229v08n01_03

Lane, M.L.S., Blum, N., & Fee, E. (2010). Oliver Wendell Holmes (1809–1894) and Ignaz Philipp Semmelweis (1818–1865): Preventing the transmission of puerperal fever. *American Journal of Public Health*, *100*(6), 1008–1009. https://doi.org/10.2105/AJPH.2009.185363

Lang, A., Ott, P., del Giudice, R., & Schabus, M. (2020). Memory traces formed in utero: Newborns' autonomic and neuronal responses to prenatal stimuli and the maternal voice. *Brain Sciences*, *10*(11), 837. https://doi.org/10.3390/brainsci10110837

Lazzerini, M., Covi, B., Mariani, I., Drglin, Z., Arendt, M., Nedberg, I.H., Elden, H., Costa, R., Drandić, D., Radetić, J., Otelea, M.R., Miani, C., Brigidi, S., Rozée, V., Ponikvar, B.M., Tasch, B., Kongslien, S., Linden, K., Barata, C., Kurbanović, M., Ružičić, J., Batram-Zantvoort, S., Castañeda, L.M., de La Rochebrochard, E., Bohinec, A., Skirnisdottir Vik, E., Zaigham, M., Santos, T., Wandschneider, L., Canales Viver, A., Ćerimagić, A., Sacks, E., & Pessa Valente, E. (2022). Quality of facility-based maternal and newborn care around the time of childbirth during the Covid-19 pandemic: Online survey investigating maternal perspectives in 12 countries of the WHO European Region. *The Lancet Regional Health – Europe*, *13*, 100268. https://doi.org/10.1016/j.lanepe.2021.100268

Leach, L.S., Poyser, C., Cooklin, A.R., & Giallo, R. (2016). Prevalence and course of anxiety disorders (and symptom levels) in men across the perinatal period: A systematic review. *Journal of Affective Disorders*, *190*, 675–686. https://doi.org/10.1016/j.jad.2015.09.063

Le Bas, G.A., Youssef, G.J., Macdonald, J.A., Rossen, L., Teague, S.J., Kothe, E.J., & Hutchinson, D.M. (2020). The role of antenatal and postnatal maternal bonding in infant development: A systematic review and meta-analysis. *Social Development*, *29*(1), 3–20, https://doi.org/10.1111/sode.12392

Lebel, C., MacKinnon, A., Bagshawe, M., Tomfohr-Madsen, L., & Giesbrecht, G. (2020). Elevated depression and anxiety symptoms among pregnant individuals during the COVID-19 pandemic. *Journal of Affective Disorders*, *277*, 5–13. https://doi.org/10.1016/j.jad.2020.07.126

Levin-Landheer, P. (1982). The cycle of development. *Transactional Analysis Journal*, *12*(2), 129–139. https://doi.org/10.1177/036215378201200207

Little, R. (1999). The shame loop: A method for working with couples. *Transactional Analysis Journal*, *29*(2), 141–148. https://doi.org/10.1177/036215379902900209

Liu, C.H., Erdei, C., & Mittal., (2021). Risk factors for depression, anxiety and PTSD symptoms in perinatal women during the COVID-19 Pandemic. *Psychiatry Research*, *295*, 113552. https://doi.org/10.1016/jpsychres.2020.113552

Lokken, E.M., Walker, C.L., Delaney, S., Kachikis, A., Kretzer, N.M., Erickson, A., Resnick, R., Vanderhoeven, J., Hwang, J.K., Barnhart, N., Rah, J., McCartney, S.A., Ma, K.K., Huebner, E.M., Thomas, J., Sheng, J.S., Paek, B.W., Retzlaff, K., Kline, C.R., Munson, J., Blain, M. LaCourse, S., Deutsch, G., & Adams Waldorf, K.M. (2020). Clinical characteristics of 46 pregnant women with a severe acute respiratory syndrome coronavirus 2 infection in Washington State. *American Journal of Obstetrics and Gynecology*, *223*(6), 911.e1–911.e14. https://doi.org/10.1016/j.ajog.2020.05.031

Lorenzer, A. (1977). *Sprachspiel und Interaktionsformen* (Language Games and Interaction Forms). Frankfurt/M: SuhrKamp.

Lorenzer, A. (1986). Tiefenhermeneutische Kulturanalyse. In Alfred Lorenzer (Ed.) *Kultur-Analysen: Psychoanalytische Studien zur Kultur* (pp. 11–98). Frankfurt/M: Fischer.

Lynch, S.H., & Lobo, M.L. (2012) Compassion fatigue in family caregivers: A Wilsonian concept analysis. *Journal of Advanced Nursing*, *68*, 2125–2134. https://doi.org/10.1111/j.1365-2648.2012.05985.x.

Lyons-Ruth, K. (1998). Implicit relational knowing: Its role in development and psychoanalytic treatment. *Infant Mental Health Journal*, *19*(3), 282–289.

Lyons-Ruth, K. (1999). The two-person unconscious: Intersubjective dialogue, enactive relational representation, and the emergence of new forms of relational organization. *Psychoanalytic Inquiry*, *19*(4), 576–617. https://doi.org/10.1080/07351699909534267

Lyons-Ruth, K., Bronfman, E., & Atwood, G. (1999). A relational diathesis model of hostile-helpless states of mind: Expressions in mother–infant interaction. In J. Solomon & C. George (Eds.), *Attachment disorganization* (pp. 33–70). New York: The Guilford Press.

Lyons-Ruth, K., & Yarger, H. (2022). Developmental costs associated with early maternal withdrawal. *Child Development Perspectives*, *16*(1), 10–17. https://doi.org/10.1111/cdep.12442

MacDonald, M. (1981). *Mystical bedlam: Madness, anxiety and healing in seventeenth-century England*. Cambridge: Cambridge University Press.

Machin, A. (2018). *The life of Dad: The making of the modern father*. London: Simon & Schuster.

MacKinnon, D.W. (1962). The nature and nurture of creative talent. *American Psychologist*, *17*(7), 484–495. https://doi.org/10.1037/h0046541

Make Mothers Matter (Maternal Health Care in the EU) (May 2021). https://makemothersmatter.org/wp-content/uploads/2021/12/2021.05.06-Maternal-Health-Care-in-the-EU-FINAL.pdf

Mancia, M. (2007). *Feeling the words: Neuropsychoanalytic understanding of memory and the unconscious* (Trans. J. Baggott). London: Routledge. (Original work published 2004)

Mansfield, A.K., Addis, M.E., & Mahalik, J.R. (2003). "Why won't he go to the doctor?" The psychology of men's help seeking. *International Journal of Men's Health, 2*(2), 93–109 www.researchgate.net/profile/James-Mahalik-2/publication/239325580_ Why_Won't_He_Go_to_the_Doctor_The_Psychology_of_Men's_Help_Seeking/ links/552401f00cf2b123c5170c7d/Why-Wont-He-Go-to-the-Doctor-The-Psychology-of-Mens-Help-Seeking.pdf

Marinho, I., Gato, J., & Coimbra, S. (2020). Parenthood intentions, pathways to parenthood, and experiences in the health services of trans people: An exploratory study in Portugal. *Sexuality Research and Social Policy, 18*, 682–692. https://doi.org/10.1007/s13178-020-00491-5

Mariño-Narvaez, C., Puertas-Gonzalez, J.A., Romero-Gonzalez, B., & Peralta-Ramirez, M.I. (2020). Giving birth during the COVID-19 pandemic: The impact on birth satisfaction and postpartum depression. *International Journal of Gynaecology & Obstetrics, 153*(1), 83–88. https://doi.org/10.1002/ijgo.1356

Marks-Tarlow, T. (2018). Awakening clinical intuition: Creativity and play. In T. Marks-Tarlow, M. Solomon, & D.J. Siegel (Eds.), *Play & Creativity in Psychotherapy*. New York: W.W. Norton.

Marland, H. (2004). *Dangerous motherhood: Insanity and childbirth in Victorian Britain*. Basingstoke: Palgrave MacMillan.

Maswime, S., & Chauke, L. (2022). Most maternal deaths are preventable: How to improve outcomes in South Africa. *The Conversation*, 4 May. https://theconversation.com/most-maternal-deaths-are-preventable-how-to-improve-outcomes-in-south-africa-181282

Matthey, S., Barnett, B., Howie, P., & Kavanagh, D.J. (2003). Diagnosing postpartum depression in mothers and fathers: Whatever happened to anxiety? *Journal of Affective Disorders, 74*(2), 139–147. https://doi.org/10.1016/s0165-0327(02)00012-5

Mayers, A., Hambridge, S., Bryant, O., & Arden-Close, E. (2020). Supporting women who develop poor postnatal mental health: What support do fathers receive to support their partner and their own mental health? *BMC Pregnancy and Childbirth, 20*(1), 359. https://doi.org.10.1186/s12884-020-03043-2

Mazza, M., Kotzalidis, G.D., Avallone, C., Balocchi, M., Sessa, I., De Luca, I., Hirsch, D., Simonetti, A., Haniri, D., Loi, E., Marano, G., Albano, G., Fasulo, V., Borghi, S., Gonsalez del Castillo A., Serio, A.M., Monti, L., Chieffo, D., Angeletti, G., Janiri, L., & Sani, G. (2022). Depressive symptoms in expecting fathers: Is paternal perinatal depression a valid concept? A systematic review of evidence. *Journal of Personalised Medicine, 12*(10), 1598. https://doi.org/10.3390/jpm12101598

MBRRACE-UK (2020). Saving lives, improving mothers' care. www.npeu.ox.ac.uk

McQuillin, J., & Welford, E. (2013). How many people are gathered here? Group work and family constellation theory. *Transactional Analysis Journal, 43*(4), 352–365. https://doi.org/10.1177/0362153713519743

McVean, A. (2017). *The history of hysteria*. Office for Science and Society, McGill University. www.mcgill.ca/oss/article/history-quackery/history-hysteria

Meager, I., Milgrom, J. (1996). Group treatment for postpartum depression: A pilot study. *Australian and New Zealand Journal of Psychiatry, 30*(6), 852–860.

Mellacqua, Z. (2021). *Transactional analysis of schizophrenia: The naked self*. London: Routledge.

Mellor, K., & Schiff, E. (1975). Discounting. *Transactional Analysis Journal, 5*(3), 295–302. https://doi.org/10.1177/036215377500500321

Meltzer-Brody, S. (2011). New insights into perinatal depression: Pathogenesis and treatment during pregnancy and postpartum. *Dialogues in Clinical Neuroscience, 13*, 89–100.

Meltzoff, A.N. (1990). Foundations for developing a concept of self: The role of imitation in relating self to other and the value of social mirroring, social modelling, and self practice in infancy, in D. Cicchetti & M. Beeghly (Eds), *The Self in Transition: Infancy to Childhood*. Chicago, IL: University of Chicago Press.

Mental Health Taskforce (2016). *The five year forward view for mental health: A report from the independent Mental Health Taskforce to the NHS in England*. www.england.nhs.uk/wp-content/uploads/2016/02/Mental-Health-Taskforce-FYFV-final.pdf

Merla, L. (2008). Determinants, costs, and meanings of Belgian stay-at-home fathers: An international comparison. *Fathering: A Journal of Theory, Research, and Practice about Men as Fathers*, 6(2), 113–132. https://doi.org/10.3149/fth.0602.113

Miller, A. (1991). *Breakdown down the wall of silence: Deliberating experience of facing painful truth*. New York: Dutton.

Milner, M. (1987a). The framed gap. In M. Milner, *The suppressed madness of sane men: Forty-four years of exploring psychoanalysis* (pp. 104–108). London: Tavistock Publications. (Original work published 1952)

Milner, M. (1987b). The role of illusion in symbol formation. In M. Milner, *The suppressed madness of sane men: Forty-four years of exploring psychoanalysis* (pp. 62–84). London: Tavistock Publications. (Original work published 1952)

Milner, M. (1987c). Winnicott and the two-way journey. In M. Milner, *The suppressed madness of sane men: Forty-four years of exploring psychoanalysis* (pp. 203–207). London: Tavistock Publications. (Original work published 1952)

Minikin, K. (2011). Transactional analysis amid the wider world: The politics and psychology of alienation. In H. Fowlie & C. Sills (Eds), *Relational transactional analysis: Principles in practice*. London: Karnac Books.

Minikin, K. (2018). Radical relational psychiatry: Toward a democracy of mind and people. *Transactional Analysis Journal*, 48(2), 111–125. https://doi.org/10.1080/03621537.2018.1429287

Minikin, K. (2020). Transactional analysis and our philosophical premises: 70 years on. *Psychotherapy and Politics International*, 18(3). https://doi.org/10.1002/ppi.1563

Minikin, K. (2021a). Treatment planning: Pathway to cure. *Transactional Analysis Journal*, 51(3), 254–266. https://doi.org/10.1080/03621537.2021.1951975

Minikin, K. (2021b). Relative privilege and the seduction of normativity. *Transactional Analysis Journal*, 51(1), 35–48. https://doi.org/10.1080/03621537.2020.1853349

Minikin, K.S. (2024). Radical-relational perspectives in transactional analysis psychotherapy: Oppression, alienation, reclamation. In *Innovations in transactional analysis: Theory and practice*. London: Routledge

Minikin, K., & Tudor, K. (2015). Gender psychopolitics: Men becoming, being and belonging. In R. Erskine (Ed.), *Transactional analysis in contemporary psychotherapy* (pp. 257–275). London: Karnac Books.

Mitchell, A.R., Gordon, H., Lindquist, A., Walker, P., Homer, C.S.E., Middleton, A., Cluver, C.A., Tong, S., & Hastie, R. (2023). Prevalence of perinatal depression in low- and middle-income countries: A systematic review and meta-analysis. *JAMA Psychiatry*, 80(5), 425–431. https://doi.org/10.1001/jamapsychiatry.2023.0069

Monk, C., Lugo-Candelas, C., & Trumpff, C. (2019). Prenatal developmental origins of future psychopathology: Mechanisms and pathways. *Annual Review of Clinical Psychology*, 15, 317–344. https://doi.org/10.1146/annurev-clinpsy-050718-095539

Moran, E., Bradshaw, C., Tuohy, T., & Noonan, M. (2021). The paternal experience of fear of childbirth: An integrative review. *International Journal of Environmental Research and Public Health*, 18(3), 1231. https://doi.org/10.3390/ijerph18031231

Moyer, C.A., Compton, S.D., Kaselitz, E., & Muzik, M. (2020). Pregnancy-related anxiety during COVID-19: A nationwide survey of 2740 pregnant women. *Archives of Women Mental Health, 23*(6), 757–765. https://doi.org/10.1007/s00737-020-01073-5

Mühleisen, T.W., Leber, M., Schulze, T.G., Strohmaier, J., Degenhardt, F., Treutlein, J., Mattheisen, M., Forstner, A.J., Schumacher, J., Breuer, R., Meier, S., Herms, S., Hoffmann, P., Lacour, A., Witt, S.H., Reif, A., Müller-Myhsok, B., Lucae, S., Maier, W., Schwarz, M., et al. (2014). Genome-wide association study reveals two new risk loci for bipolar disorder. *Nature Communications. 11*(5), 3339.

Mulkey, S.B., & Plessis, A.D. (2018). The critical role of the central autonomic nervous system in fetal-neonatal transition. *Seminars in Pediatric Neurology*, 28, 29–37. https://doi.org/10.1016/j.spen.2018.05.004

Munk-Olsen, T., Maegbaek, M.L., Johannsen, B.M., Liu, X., Howard, L.M., di Florio, A., Bergink, V., & Meltzer-Brody, S. (2016). Perinatal psychiatric episodes: A population-based study on treatment incidence and prevalence. *Translational Psychiatry*, 6(10), e919. https://doi.org/10.1038/tp.2016.190

Nakku, J.E., Okello, E.S., Kizza, D., Honikman, S., Ssebunnya, J., Ndyanabangi, S., Hanlon, C., & Kigozi, F. (2016). Perinatal mental health care in a rural African district, Uganda: A qualitative study of barriers, facilitators and needs. *BMC Health Service Research*, 16, 295. https://doi.org/10.1186/s12913-016-1547-7

Nationwide Children's Hospital (2023). Family resources & education, health, wellness and safety resources, helping hands, infant vision birth to one year. www.nationwidechildrens.org/family-resources-education/health-wellness-and-safety-resources/helping-hands/infant-vision-birth-to-one-year#:~:text=One%20week%20after%20birth%2C%20your,see%20about%2012%20inches%20away

Neugebauer, C., Oh, W., McCarty, M., & Mastergeorge, A.M. (2022). Mother–infant dyadic synchrony in the NICU context. *Advances in Neonatal Care: Official Journal of the National Association of Neonatal Nurses, 22*(2), 170–179. https://doi.org/10.1097/ANC.000000000000085

Norcross, J.C., & Guy, J.D.J. (2007). *Leaving it at the office: A guide to psychotherapist self-care* (Adobe Digital Editions version). https://ebookcentral.proquest.com

Novak, E.T. (2013). Combining traditional ego state theory and relational approaches to transactional analysis in working with trauma and dissociation. *Transactional Analysis Journal, 43*(3), 186–196. https://doi.org/10.1177/0362153713509952

Novak, E.T. (2022). Emancipation from a fear of institutionalization: A case study of transgenerational hauntings. *Transactional Analysis Journal, 52*(2), 106–119. https://doi.org/10.1080/03621537.2022.2044112

O'Brien, A.P., McNeil, K.A., Fletcher, R., Conrad, A., Wilson, A.J., Jones, D., & Chan, S.W. (2017). New fathers' perinatal depression and anxiety – treatment options: An integrative review. *American Journal of Men's Health, 11*(4), 863–876. https://doi.org/10.1177/1557988316669047

Odinka, P., Odinka, J., Ezeme, M., Ndukuba, A., Amadi, K., Muomah, R., et al. (2019). Socio-demographic correlates of postpartum psychological distress among apparently healthy mothers in two tertiary hospitals in Enugu, South-East Nigeria. *Africa Health Sciences, 19*(3), 2515–2525.

O'Dwyer, D. (2017). *A psychotherapeutic exploration of the effects of absent fathers on children*. Thesis submitted in partial fulfilment of the requirements of the BA Counselling and Psychotherapy Department of Psychotherapy, Dublin Business School, School of Arts, 2 May 2017.

OECD (2021). Family database in the Asia-Pacific region OECD and OECD KOREA Policy Centre. LMF1.4: *Employment profiles over the life-course.* Updated December 2021. https://oecdkorea.org/resource/download/2022/kor/LMF_1_4_Employment_profiles_over_life_course_2021.pdf

OECD (2022). *OECD statistics, health status: Maternal and infant mortality.* https:// stats.oecd.org/index.aspx?queryid=30116

Ogden, T.H. (2012). *Creative readings: Essays on seminal analytic works.* London and New York: Routledge.

O'Hara, M.W., & McCabe, J.E. (2013). Postpartum depression: Current status and future directions. *Annual Review of Clinical Psychology, 9,* 379–407.

O'Mahen, H.A., Grieve, H., Jones, J., McGinley, J., Woodford, J., & Wilkinson, E. (2015). Women's experiences of factors affecting treatment engagement and adherence in internet delivered behavioural activation for postnatal depression. *Internet Interventions, 2*(1), 84–90. https://doi.org/10.1016/j.invent.2014.11.003

Omeish, Y., & Kiernan, S. (2020). Targeting bias to improve maternal care and outcomes for Black women in the USA. *EClinicalMedicine, 27,* 100568. https://doi. org/10.1016/j.eclinm.2020.100568

ONS (Office for National Statistics) (2022a). *Families and the labour market, UK: 2021.* https://backup.ons.gov.uk/wp-content/uploads/sites/3/2022/07/Families-and-the-labour-market-UK-2021.pdf

ONS (Office for National Statistics) (2022b). *Census 2021. Who are the children entering care in England?* Office For National Statistics, Data and analysis from Census 2021. www.ons.gov.uk/peoplepopulationandcommunity/healthandsocialcare/ socialcare/articles/whoarethechildrenenteringcareinengland/2022-11-04

PAHO (Pan American Health Organization) (2023). *PAHO and partners launch campaign to reduce maternal mortality in Latin America and the Caribbean.* www. paho.org/en/news/8-3-2023-paho-and-partners-launch-campaign-reduce-maternal-mortality-latin-america-and#:~:text=Last%20year%2C%20the%20maternal%20 mortality,68%20per%20100%2C000%20live%20births

Palmér, L. (2019). Previous breastfeeding difficulties: An existential breastfeeding trauma with two intertwined pathways for future breastfeeding – fear and longing. *International Journal of Qualitative Studies in Health and Well-being, 14*(1). https:// doi.org/10.1080/17482631.2019.1588034

Parkin, F. (2014). Breaking the circuit: The power of empathy and understanding interlocking racket systems in deepening work with couples. *Transactional Analysis Journal, 44*(3), 208–217. https://doi.org/10.1177/0362153714550983

Patton, G.C., Romaniuk, H., Spry, E., Coffey, C., Olsson, C., Doyle, L.W., Oats, J., Hearps, S., Carlin, J.B., & Brown, S. (2015). Prediction of perinatal depression from adolescence and before conception (VIHCS): 20-year prospective cohort study. *Lancet, 386*(9996), 875–883. https://doi.org/10.1016/S0140-6736(14)62248-0

Paulson, J.F., & Bazemore, S.D. (2010). Prenatal, postpartum depression in fathers its association with maternal depression: a meta-analysis. *JAMA, 303,* 1961–1969. https://doi.org/10.1001/jama.2010.605

Piaget, J. (1952). *The origins of intelligence in the child.* New York: International University Press.

Piaget, J. (1962). *Play, dreams, and imitation in childhood.* New York: W.W. Norton.

Pierini, A. (2008). Has the unconscious moved house? *Transactional Analysis Journal, 38*(2), 110–118. https://doi.org/10.1177/036215370803800204

Pilav, S., Easter, A., Silverio, S.A., De Backer, K., Sundaresh, S., Roberts, S., Howard, L.M. (2022). Experiences of perinatal mental health care among minority ethnic women during the COVID-19 pandemic in London: A qualitative study. *International Journal of Environmental Research and Public Health, 19*(4), 1975. https://doi. org/10.3390/ijerph19041975

Pollack, L.M., Chen, J., Cox, S., Luo, F., Robbins, C.L., Tevendale, H.D., Li, R., & Ko, J.Y. (2022). Healthcare utilization and costs associated with perinatal depression among Medicaid enrollees. *American Journal of Preventive Medicine*, *62*(6), e333–e341. https://doi.org/10.1016/j.amepre.2021.12.008

Porges, S.W. (2011). *The polyvagal theory: Neurophysiological foundations of emotions, attachment, communication, and self-regulation*. New York: W.W. Norton.

Pouba, K.T., & Tianen, A. (2006). Lunacy in the 19th century: Women's admission to asylums in United States of America. *Oshkosh Scholar*, *1*, 95–103.

Power, R.A., Tansey, K.E., Buttenschøn, H.N., Cohen-Woods, S., Bigdeli, T., Hall, L.S., Kutalik, Z., Lee, S.H., Ripke, S., Steinberg, S., Teumer, A., Viktorin, A., Wray, N.R., Arolt, V., Baune, B.T., Boomsma, D.I., Børglum, A.D., Byrne, E.M., Castelao, E., Craddock, N. et al. (2017). Genome-wide association for major depression through age at onset stratification: Major Depressive Disorder Working Group of the Psychiatric Genomics Consortium, *Biological Psychiatry*, *81*(4), 325–335, https://doi.org/10.1016/j.biopsych.2016.05.010; www.sciencedirect.com/science/article/pii/S0006322316323861

Primack, J.M., Addis, M.E., Syzdek, M., & Miller, I.W. (2010). The men's stress workshop: A gender-sensitive treatment for depressed men. *Cognitive and Behavioral Practice*, *17*, 77–87. https://doi.org/10.1016/j.cbpra.2009.07.002

Psouni, E., Frisk, C., & Brocki, K. (2021). Anxiety among fathers in the postnatal period: Links to depression, attachment insecurity and emotion regulation. *Journal of Affective Disorders Reports*, *6*. https://doi.org/10.1016/j.jadr.100276

Rallis, S., Skouteris, H., McCabe, M., & Milgrom, J. (2014). The transition to motherhood: Towards a broader understanding of perinatal distress. *Women and Birth*, *27*, 68–71.

Ramchandani, P., O'Connor, T., Evans, J., Heron, J., Murray, L., & Stein, A. (2008). The effects of pre- and postnatal depression in fathers: A natural experiment comparing the effects of exposure to depression on offspring. *Journal of Child Psychology and Psychiatry*, *49*(10), 1069–1078. https://doi.org/10.1111/j.1469-7610.2008.02000.x

Ramchandani, P., Stein, A., Evans, J., & O'Connor, T. (2005). Paternal depression in the postnatal period and child development: a prospective population study. *Lancet*, *365*(9478), 2201–2205. Https://doi.org/10.1016/S0140-6736(05)66778-5

Read, J., Lewis, S., Horowitz, M., & Moncrieff, J. (2023). The need for antidepressant withdrawal support services: Recommendations from 708 patients. *Psychiatry Research*, *326*, 115303. https://doi.org/10.1016/j.psychres.2023.115303

Reddy, V., & Trevarthen, C. (2004). What we learn about babies from engaging their emotions. *Zero to Three*, *24*(3), 9–15.

Ritter, S.M., Damian, R.I., Simonton, D.K., van Baaren, R.B., Strick, M., Derks, J., & Dijksterhuis, A. (2012). Diversifying experiences enhance cognitive flexibility. *Journal of Experimental Social Psychology*, *48*(4), 961–964. https://doi.org/10.1016/j.jesp.2012.02.009.

Ritter, S.M., & Dijksterhuis, A. (2014). Creativity: The unconscious foundations of the incubation period. *Frontiers in Human Neuroscience*, *8*, Article 215. https://doi.org/10.3389/fnhum.2014.00215

Ritter, S.M., Gu, X., Crijns, M., & Biekens, P. (2020). Fostering students' creative thinking skills by means of a one-year creativity training program. *PLoS One*, *15*(3), e0229773. https//doi.org/10.1371/journal.pone.0229773

Rochat, P. (2003). Five levels of self-awareness as they unfold early in life. *Consciousness & Cognition*, *12*, 717–731. https://doi.org/10.1016/S1053-8100(03)00081-3

Rochat, P., (2009). *Others in mind: Social origins of self-consciousness*. Cambridge: Cambridge University Press.

Rominov, H., Giallo, R., Pilkington, P., & Whelan, T. (2018). "Getting help for yourself is a way of helping your baby": Fathers' experiences of support for mental health and parenting in the perinatal period. *Psychology of Men & Masculinities, 19*(3), 457–468. https://doi.org/10.1037/men0000103

Rowe, H.J., Holton, S., & Fisher, J.R. (2013). Postpartum emotional support: A qualitative study of women's and men's anticipated needs and preferred sources. *Australian Journal of Primary Health, 19*(1), 46–52. https://doi.org/10.1071/PY11117

Royal College of Midwives (RCM) (2021). Media release "Value NHS staff and invest in them" says Royal College of Midwives responding to CQC State of Care report published 22 October by the Royal College of Midwives.

Rublein, L., & Muschalla, B. (2022). Childbirth fear, birth-related mindset and knowledge in non-pregnant women without birth experience. *BMC Pregnancy and Childbirth, 22*(1), 249. https://doi.org/10.1186/s12884-022-04582-6

Sabin, J.A. (2020). How we fail black patients in pain. *AAMC.ORG Viewpoints.* www.aamc.org/news/how-we-fail-black-patients-pain

Safran, J.D., Muran, J.C., & Eubanks-Carter, C. (2011). Repairing alliance ruptures. *Psychotherapy, 48*(1), 80–87. https://doi.org/10.1037/a0022140

Salary.com (2019). *How much is a mother really worth?* www.salary.com/articles/mother-salary/

SANDS (2021). Baby loss and pregnancy loss statistics. SANDS, UK. www.sands.org.uk/how-many-babies-die-uk

Scilligo, P. (2009). *Transazionale socio-cognitive* [Social-cognitive transactional analysis]. Rome: LAS.

Scilligo, P. (2011). Transference as a measurable social-cognitive process: An application of Scilligo's model of ego states. *Transactional Analysis Journal, 41*, 196–205.

Schiff, A.W., & Schiff, J.L. (1971). Passivity. *Transactional Analysis Journal, 1*(1), 71–78. https://doi.org/10.1177/036215377100100114

Schizophrenia Working Group of the Psychiatric Genomics Consortium (2014). Biological insights from 108 schizophrenia-associated genetic loci. *Nature, 511*, 421–427. https://doi.org/10.1038/nature13595

Schore, A. (1994). *Affect regulation and the origin of the self. The neurobiology of emotional development.* Hillsdale, NJ: Lawrence Erlbaum.

Schore, A. (2019). *Right brain psychotherapy.* New York: W.W. Norton.

Schwarz, N., & Clore, G.L. (2007). Feelings and phenomenal experiences. In A. Kruglanski, and E.T. Higgins (Eds), *Social psychology: Handbook of basic principles.* New York: Guilford Press.

Scott, G., Lertiz, L.E., & Mumford, M.D. (2004). The effectiveness of creativity training: A quantitative review. *Creativity Research Journal, 16*(4), 361–388. https://doi.org/10.1080/10400410409534549

Shafer, K., & Renick, A.J. (2020). Depressive symptoms and father involvement in Canada: Evidence from a national study. *Canadian Review of Sociology, 57*(2), 197–222. https://doi.org/10.1111/cars.12277. Epub 17 May 2020.

Shepherd, T. (2023). Maternity crisis: Pregnant women left in despair as facilities disappear in regional Australia. *The Guardian,* 26 February. www.theguardian.com/australia-news/2023/feb/27/maternity-crisis-pregnant-women-left-in-despair-as-facilities-disappear-in-regional-australia

Shibli-Kometiani, M., Brown, A.M. (2013). Fathers' experiences accompanying labour and birth. *British Journal of Midwifery, 20*(5), 339–344. https://doi.org/10.12968/bjom.2012.20.5.339

Singley, D., & Edwards, L. (2015). Men's perinatal mental health in the transition to fatherhood. *Professional Psychology: Research And Practice, 46*(5), 309–316. https://doi.org/10.1037/pro0000032

Slade, P., Morrell, C.J., Rigby, A., Ricci, K., Spittlehouse, J., & Brugha, T.S. (2010). Postnatal women's experiences of management of depressive symptoms: A qualitative study. *British Journal of General Practice, 60*(580), e440–448. https://doi. org/10.3399/bjgp10X532611

Smythe, K.L., Petersen, I., & Schartau, P. (2022). Prevalence of perinatal depression and anxiety in both parents: A systematic review and meta-analysis. *JAMA Network Open – Original Investigation/Psychiatry, 5*(6):e2218969. https://doi.org/10.1001/ jamanetworkopen.2022.18969

Smyth, E., & Russell, H. (2021). Fathers and children from infancy to middle child-hood. *Economic & Social Research Institute*, Research Series 130. https://doi.org/ 10.26504/rs130

Snipe, M. (2022). Clinicians dismiss black women's pain. The consequences are dire. *Capital B News.* https://capitalbnews.org/black-women-pain/

Solomon, C.R. (2017). "A daddy in a mommy world": Social networks and commu-nity. In *The lives of stay-at-home fathers* (pp. 75–97). Leeds, UK: Emerald Publish-ing. https://doi.org/10.1108/978-1-78743-501-820171007

Somers-Smith, M.J. (1999). A place for the partner? Expectations and experiences of support during childbirth. *Midwifery, 15*(2), 101–108. https://doi.org/10.1016/ s0266-6138(99)90006-2

Sørensen, A., Juhl Jørgensen, K., & Munkholm, K. (2022). Clinical practice guideline recommendations on tapering and discontinuing antidepressants for depression: A systematic review. *Therapeutic Advances in Psychopharmacology, 11*(12). https://doi. org/10.1177/20451253211067656

Spratt, E.G., Marsh, C., Wahlquist, A.E., Papa, C.E., Nietert, P.J., Brady, K.T., Herbert, T.L., & Wagner, C. (2016). Biologic effects of stress and bonding in mother–infant pairs. *International Journal of Psychiatry in Medicine, 51*(3), 246–257. https://doi.org/10.1177/0091217416652382

Staneva, A., Bogossian, F, Pritchard, M., & Wittkowski, A. (2015). The effects of maternal depression, anxiety, and perceived stress during pregnancy on preterm birth: A systematic review. *Women Birth, 28*(3), 179–193. https://doi.org/10.1016/j. wombi.2015.02.003. Epub March 9 2015.

Statistic Research Department (2023). Maternal mortality rates in Russia from 2000 to 2022 (per 100,000 live births). Published by Statistic Research Department 20 July 2023.

Statistics Canada (2019). *Maternal mental health in Canada, 2018–2019.* www150. statcan.gc.ca/n1/daily-quotidien/190624/dq190624b-eng.htm#

Statistics South Africa (2022). *Maternal mortality rate on the decline in SA.* www. statssa.gov.za/?p=15321#:~:text=Nationally%2C%20the%20ratio%20decreased%20 from,experiencing%20a%20decrease%20in%20MMFR

Stechler, G., & Latz, E. (1966). Some observations on attention and arousal in the human infant. *Journal of the American Academy Child and Adolescent Psychiatry, 5*, 517–525.

Steere, D. (1981). Body movement in ego states. *Transactional Analysis Journal, 11*(4), 335–345. https://doi.org/10.1177/036215378101100418

Stellenberg, E.L., & Abrahams, J.M. (2015). Prevalence of and factors influencing postnatal depression in a rural community in South Africa. *African Journal of Pri-mary Health Care & Family Medicine, 7*(1), 874. https://doi.org/10.4102/phcfm. v7i1.874

Stern, D. (1977). *The first relationship: Infant and mother.* Cambridge, MA: Harvard University Press.

Stern, D. (1985). *The interpersonal world of the infant: A View from psychoanalysis and developmental psychology.* New York: Basic Books.

Stern, D. (2005). Intersubjectivity. In E.S. Person, A.M. Cooper, & G.O. Gabbard (Eds.), *The American psychiatric publishing textbook of psychoanalysis* (pp. 77–92). American Psychiatric Publishing.

Stern, D., Sander, L., Nahum, J., Harrison, A., Lyons-Ruth, K., Morgan, B., & Tronick, E. (1998). Non-interpretative mechanisms in psychoanalytic therapy: The "something more" than interpretation. *International Journal of Psycho-Analysis*, 79(5), 903–921.

Stilman, R. (2009) Post natal depression and the implicit client: An inclusive approach. *International Journal of Psychotherapy*, 13(2), 44–52.

Stone, A. (2019). *Being born: Birth and philosophy*. London: Oxford University Press.

Studzińska, M., Zaręba, K., Kawa, N., & Matuszyk, D. (2022). Tokophobia and anxiety in pregnant women during the SARS-CoV-2 pandemic in Poland: A prospective cross-sectional study. *International Journal of Environmental and Research and Public Health*, 19(2), 714. https://doi.org/10.3390/ijerph19020714

Stuthridge, J., & Rowland, H. (2019). Letter from the coeditors. *Transactional Analysis Journal*, 49(4), 229–232. https://doi.org/10.1080/03621537.2019.1650225

Sullivan, O. (2006). *Changing gender relations, changing families: Tracing the pace of change over time*. Boulder, CO: Rowman & Littlefield.

Sundelin, H.E., Stephansson, O., Hultman, C.M., & Ludvigsson, J.F. (2018). Pregnancy outcomes in women with autism: A nationwide population-based cohort study. *Clinical Epidemiology*, 10, 1817–1826. https://doi.org/10.2147/CLEP.S176910

Suzuki, E., Kouame, C., & Mills, S. (2003). *Progress in reducing maternal mortality has stagnated and we are not on track to achieve the SDG target: new UN report*. blogs.worldbank.org. https://blogs.worldbank.org/opendata/progress-reducing-maternal-mortality-has-stagnated-and-we-are-not-track-achieve-sdg-target

Syed, M. (2015). *Black box thinking: Yhe surprising truth about success*. London: John Murray Press.

Tai, D.B.G., Sia, I.G., Doubeni, C.A., & Wieland, M.L. (2021). Disproportionate impact of COVID-19 on racial and ethnic minority groups in the United States: A 2021 update. *Journal of Racial and Ethnic Health Disparities*, 9, 2334–2339. https://doi.org/10.1007/s40615-021-01170-w

Taipale, J. (2016). Self-regulation and beyond: Affect regulation and the infant–caregiver dyad. *Frontiers in Psychology* 7. www.frontiersin.org/journals/psychology/articles/10.3389/fpsyg.2016.00889

Tasca, C., Rapetti, M., Carta, M.G., & Fadda, B. (2012). Women and hysteria in the history of mental health. *Clinical Practice & Epidemiology in Mental Health*, 8, 110–119. https://doi.org/10.2174/1745017901208010110. Epub October 19 2012.

Tasker, F., & Gato, J. (2020). Gender identity and future thinking about parenthood: A qualitative analysis of focus group data with transgender and non-binary people in the United Kingdom. *Frontiers in Psychology*, 6(11), 865. https://doi.com/10.3389/fpsyg.2020.00865

Tauqeer, F., Ceulemans, M., Gerbier, E., Passier, A., Oliver, A., Foulon, V., Panchaud, A., Lupattelli, A., & Nordeng, H. (2023). Mental health of pregnant and postpartum women during the third wave of the COVID-19 pandemic: A European cross-sectional study. *BMJ Open*, 13(1), e063391. https://doi.org/10.1136/bmjopen-2022-063391

Thériault, A., Gazzola, N., Isenor, J., & Pascal, L. (2015). Imparting self-care practices to therapists: What the experts recommend. *Canadian Journal of Counselling and Psychotherapy*, 49(4), 389–400. https://cjc-rcc.ucalgary.ca/article/view/61031/2765-R

Tikkanen, R., Gunja, M.Z., FitzGerald, M., & Zephyrin, L. (2020). Maternal mortality and maternity care in the United States compared to 10 other developed countries. *The Commonwealth Fund*. www.commonwealthfund.org/publications/issue-briefs/2020/nov/maternal-mortality-maternity-care-us-compared-10-countries

Tilney, T. (1998). *Dictionary of transactional analysis*. London: Whurr Publishers.

Totschnig, W. (2017). Arendt's notion of natality: An attempt at clarification. *Ideas y Valores*, 66. https://doi.org/10.15446/ideasyvalores.v66n165.55202

Trawalter, S. (2022). *Black Americans are systematically under-treated for pain. Why?* Frank Batten School of Leadership and Public Policy, University of Virginia. https://batten.virginia.edu/about/news/black-americans-are-systematically-under-treated-pain-why

Tronick, E.Z. (2007). *The neurobehavioral and social emotional development of infants and children.* New York: W.W. Norton.

Tronick, E.Z., Als, H., Adamslon, L., Wise, S., & Brazelton, T.B. (1978). The infant's response to entrapment between contradictory messages in face-to-face interaction. *Journal of the American Academy of Child & Adolescent Psychiatry, 17,* 1–13. https://doi.org/10.1016/s0002-7138(09)62273-1

Tudor, K. (2010). Turning over "the relational". *European Journal of Psychotherapy & Counselling, 12*(3), 257–267. https://dx.doi.org/10.1080/13642537.2010.518439

Tustin, F. (1991). Revised understanding of psychogenic autism. *International Journal of Psychoanalysis, 72,* 585–591.

Tyer-Viola, L.A., & Lopez, R.P. (2014). Pregnancy with chronic illness. *Journal of Obstetric, Gynecologic & Neonatal Nursing, Research, 43*(1), 25–37. https://doi.org/10.1111/1552-6909.12275

United Nations Population Fund (UNFPA) (2021). *Global shortage of 900,000 midwives threatens women's lives and health, new report shows.* www.unfpa.org/news/global-shortage-900000-midwives-threatens-womens-lives-and-health-new-report-shows

UN, Yemen (2023). *After eight years of conflict and despite a fragile truce, childbirth still a matter of life and death in Yemen.* https://yemen.un.org/en/226024-after-eight-years-conflict-and-despite-fragile-truce-childbirth-still-matter-life-and-death#:~:text=A%20maternal%20health%20crisis&text=Some%205.5%20million%20women%20and,and%20childbirth%20every%20two%20hours

Val, A., Míguez, M.C. (2023). Prevalence of antenatal anxiety in European women: A literature review. *International Journal of Environmental Research and Public Health, 20*(2), 1098. https://doi.org/10.3390/ijerph20021098

Van der Gaag, N., Heilman, B., Gupta, T., Nembhard, C., & Barker, G. (2019). *State of the world's fathers: Unlocking the power of men's care.* Washington, DC: Promundo-US.

Van IJzendoorn, M.H., Schuengel, C., & Bakermans-Kranenburg, M.J. (1999). Disorganized attachment in early childhood: Meta-analysis of precursors, concomitants and sequelae. *Development and Psychopathology, 11*(2), 225–249. https://doi.org/10.1017/s0954579499002035

Visser, G.H.A., Ayres-de-Campos, D., Barnea, E.R., de Bernis, L., Di Renzo, G.C., Vidarte, M.F.E., Lloyd, I., Nassar, A.H., Nicholson, W., Shah, P.K., Stones, W., Sun, L., Theron, G.B., & Walani, S. (2018). FIGO position paper: How to stop the caesarean section epidemic. *Lancet, 392*(10155), 1286–1287. https://doi.org/10.1016/S0140-6736(18)32113-5

Wagner, P. (1993). *A sociology of modernity: Liberty and discipline.* New York and London: Routledge.

Wall, S., & Dempsey, M. (2023). The effect of COVID-10 lockdowns on women's perinatal mental health: A systematic review. *Women and Birth, 36*(1), 47–55. https://doi.org/10.1016/j.wombi.2022.06.05

Ware, P. (1983). Personality adaptations: (Doors to therapy). *Transactional Analysis Journal, 13*(1), 11–19. https://doi.org/10.1177/036215378301300104

Weinberg, M.K., Beeghly, M., Olson, K.L., & Tronick, E. (2008). A still-face paradigm for young children: 2 ½ year-olds' reactions to maternal unavailability during the still-face. *Journal of Developmental Processes, 3*(1), 4–22. www.ncbi.nlm.nih.gov/pmc/articles/PMC3289403/

Weinstein, A.D. (2016). *Prenatal development and parents' lived experiences: How early events shape our psychophysiology and relationships.* New York: W.W. Norton.

White House (2022). *White House blueprint for addressing the maternal health crisis.* www.whitehouse.gov/wp-content/uploads/2022/06/Maternal-Health-Blueprint.pdf

White House Briefing Room (2022), *Speeches and remarks: Remarks by Vice President Harris on the Administration's commitment to improve maternal health,* 21 April. www.whitehouse.gov/briefing-room/speeches-remarks/2022/04/21/remarks-by-vice-president-harris-on-the-administrations-commitment-to-improve-maternal-health/

Widdowson, M. (2010). *Transactional analysis: 100 key points & techniques.* Hove, UK: Routledge.

Wierckx, K., Van Caenegem, E., Pennings, G., Elaut, E., Dedecker, D., Van de Peer, F., Weyers, S., De Sutter, P., & T'Sjoen, G. (2012). Reproductive wish in transsexual men. *Human Reproduction, 27*(2), 483–487. https://doi.com/10.1093/humrep/der406. Epub 28 November 2011.

Williamson, M.T. (1987) Sex differences in depression symptoms among adult family medicine patients. *Journal of Family Practice, 25,* 591–594.

Winkler, D., Pjrek, E., & Kasper, S. (2005). Anger attacks in depression: Evidence for a male depressive syndrome. *Psychotherapy and Psychosomatics, 74,* 303–307. https://doi.org/10.1159/000086321

Winnicott, D.W. (1953). Transitional objects and transitional phenomena. *International Journal of Psychoanalysis, 34,* 89–97.

Winnicott, D.W. (1956/1984). Primary maternal preoccupation. In *Through paediatrics to psychoanalysis: Collected papers* (pp. 300–305). London: Karnac.

Winnicott, D.W. (1960). The theory of the parent–infant relationship. *International Journal of Psychoanalysis, 41,* 585–595.

Winnicott, D.W. (1963). From dependence towards independence in the development of the individual. In D.W. Winnicott (Ed., 1990), *The maturational processes and the facilitating environment* (pp. 83–92). London: Karnac.

Winnicott, D.W. (1971). *Playing and reality.* London: Tavistock Publications.

Winnicott, D.W. (2005 [1971]). *Playing and reality.* London: Routledge.

Wisner, K.L., Sit, D.K.Y., McShea, M.C., Rizzo, D.M., Zoertich, R.A., Hughes, C.L., Eng, H.F., Luther, J.F., Wisniewski, S.R., Costantino, M.L., Confer, A.L., Moses-Kolko, E.L., Famy, C.S., & Hanusa, B.H. (2013). Onset timing, thoughts of self-harm, and diagnoses in postpartum women with screen-positive depression findings. *JAMA Psychiatry, 70*(5), 490–498. https://doi.org/10.1001/jamapsychiatry.2013.87

Wolf, J.B., & Wade, M.J. (2009). What are maternal effects (and what are they not)? *Philosophical Transactions of the Royal Society of London. Series B, Biological sciences, 364*(1520), 1107–1115. https://doi.org/10.1098/rstb.2008.0238

Wolff, P. (1966). The causes, controls, and organization of behaviour in the neonate. *Psychological Issues, 5*(1), 1–105.

Woodhead, S., Marley, C., Calia, C., Guerra, C., Reid, C., Burke, J.P., & Amos, A. (2023). Maternal mental health in Sub-Saharan Africa: A systematic review of interventions for common perinatal mental health disorders. *Research Square.* https://doi.org/10.21203/rs.3.rs-2769632/v1

Woody, C.A., Ferrari, A.J., Siskind, D.J., Whiteford, H.A., & Harris, M.G. (2017). A systematic review and meta-regression of the prevalence and incidence of perinatal depression. *Journal of Affective Disorders, 219,* 86–92. https://doi.10.1016/j.jad.2017.05.003

World Bank (2022a). *Number of maternal deaths: Sub-Saharan Africa.* https://data.worldbank.org/indicator/SH.MMR.DTHS?locations=ZG

World Bank (2022b). *Female labor force participation. Source: International Labour Organization (ILO).* World Bank Gender Data Portal. https://genderdata.worldbank.org/data-stories/flfp-data-story/

World Health Organization (WHO) (2016a). *Mental health determinants and populations: Department of Mental Health and Substance Dependence. Maternal and child mental health program.* www.who.int/mental_health/maternal-child/maternal_mental_health/en/

World Health Oranization (WHO) (2016b). *mhGAO intervention guide for mental, neurological and substance use disorders in non-specialized health settings: Mental health Gap Action Programme (mhGAP).* Geneva: World Health Organization.

World Health Organization (WHO) (2018). *Nurturing care for early childhood development: A framework for helping children survive and thrive to transform health and human potential.* Geneva: World Health Organization.

World Health Organization (WHO) (2022). *Launch of the WHO guide for integration of perinatal mental health in maternal and child health services.* www.who.int/news/item/19-09-2022-launch-of-the-who-guide-for-integration-of-perinatal-mental-health#:~:text=Almost%201%20in%205%20women,undertake%20acts%20of%20self%2Dharm

World Health Organization (WHO) (2023). *Family planning, contraception methods.* www.who.int/news-room/fact-sheets/detail/family-planning-contraception

Yakupova, V., & Suarez, A. (2022). Postpartum PTSD and birth experience in Russian-speaking women. *Midwifery, 112,* 103385. https://doi.org/10.1016/j.midw.2022.103385. Epub 27 May 2022.

Yan, H., Ding, Y., & Guo, W. (2020). Mental health of pregnant and postpartum women during the Coronavirus disease 2019 pandemic: A systematic review and meta-analysis. *Frontiers in Psychology, 30,* e36. https://doi.org/10.1017/S2045796021000275

Yang, X., Fang, Y., Chen, H., Zhang, T., Yin, X., Man, J., Yang, L., & Lu, M. (2021). Global, regional and national burden of anxiety disorders from 1990 to 2019: Results from the Global Burden of Disease Study 2019. *Epidemiology and Psychiatric Sciences, 30,* e36. https://doi.org/10.1017/S2045796021000275

Zeanah, C.H., Danis, B., Hirshberg, L., Benoit, D., Miller, D., & Heller, S.S. (1999). Disorganized attachment associated with partner violence: A research note. *Infant Mental Health Journal, 20*(1), 77–86. https://doi.org/10.1002/(SICI)1097-0355(199921)20:1<77::AID-IMHJ6>3.0.CO;2-S

Yousaf, O., Popat, A., & Hunter, M.S. (2015). An investigation of masculinity attitudes, gender, and attitudes toward psychological help-seeking. *Psychology of Men and Masculinity, 16*(2), 234–237. https://doi.org/10.1037/a0036241

INDEX

Note: Locators in *italic* indicate figures and in **bold** tables.